THE CURE FOR HICCUPS

Written and illustrated by Todd Remonda

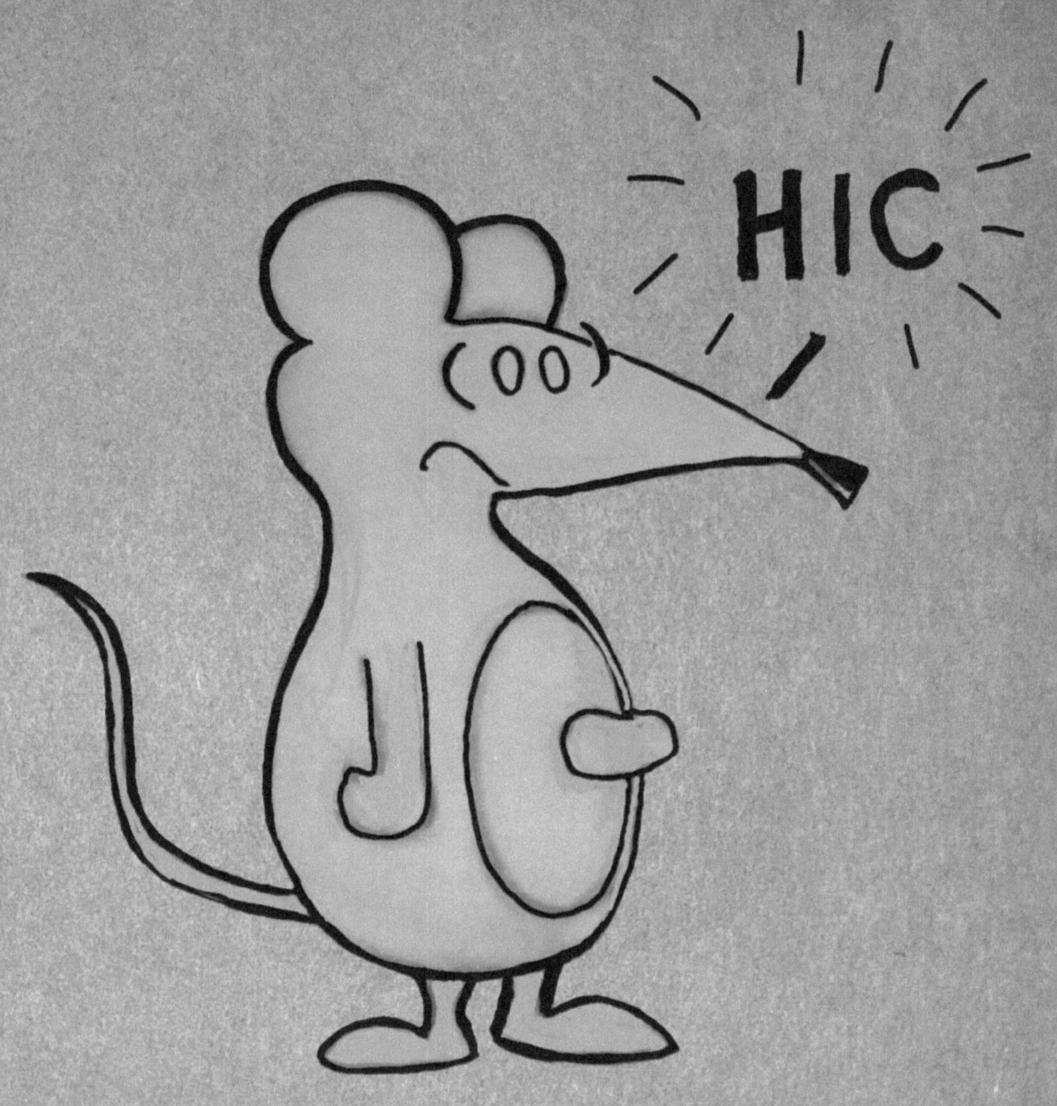

(oo)
HIC

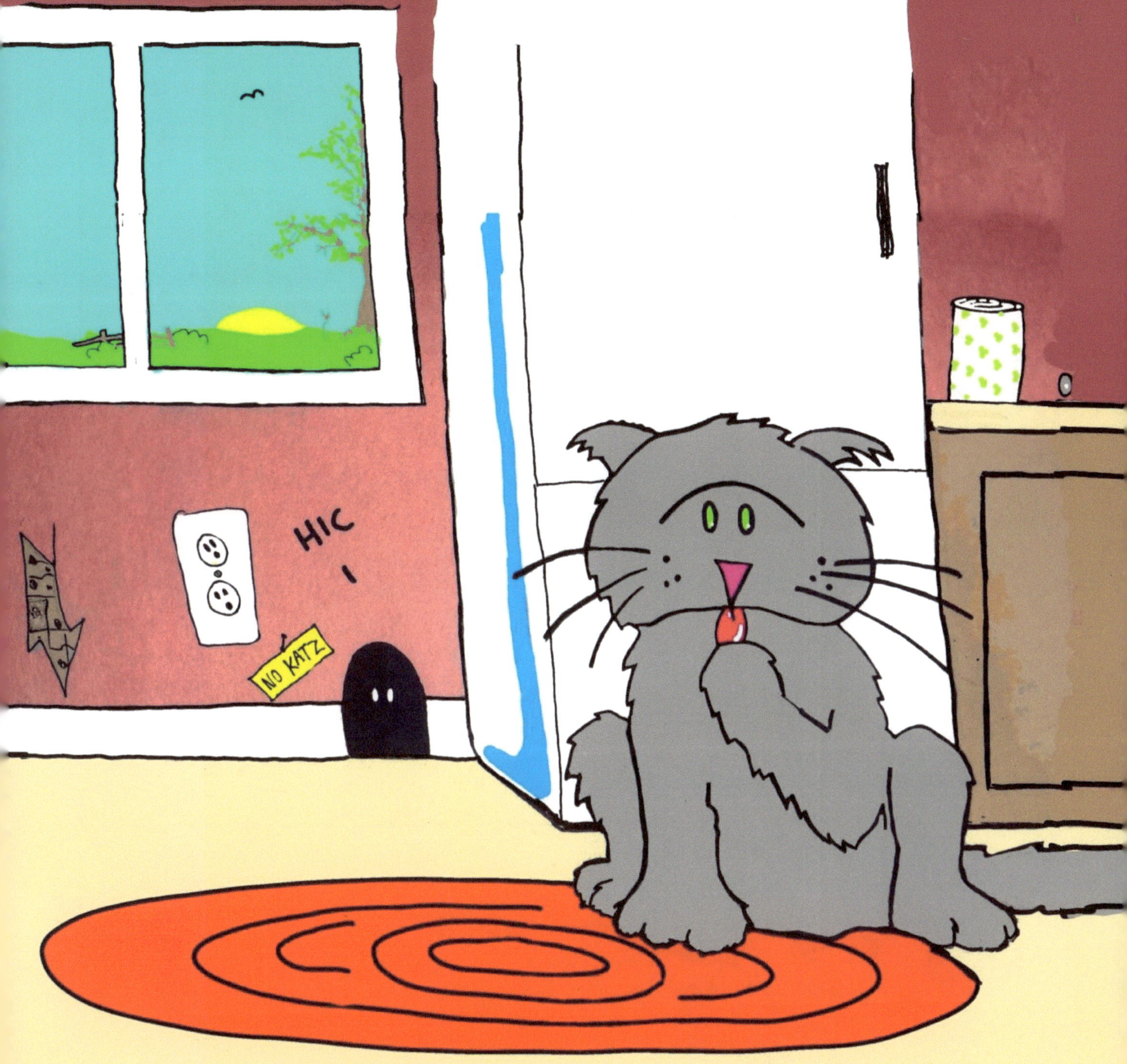

Tommy the mouse had a problem or two.
He had hiccups all night and didn't know what to do!

Dad, tired and grumpy, said,
"Stop that right now!"

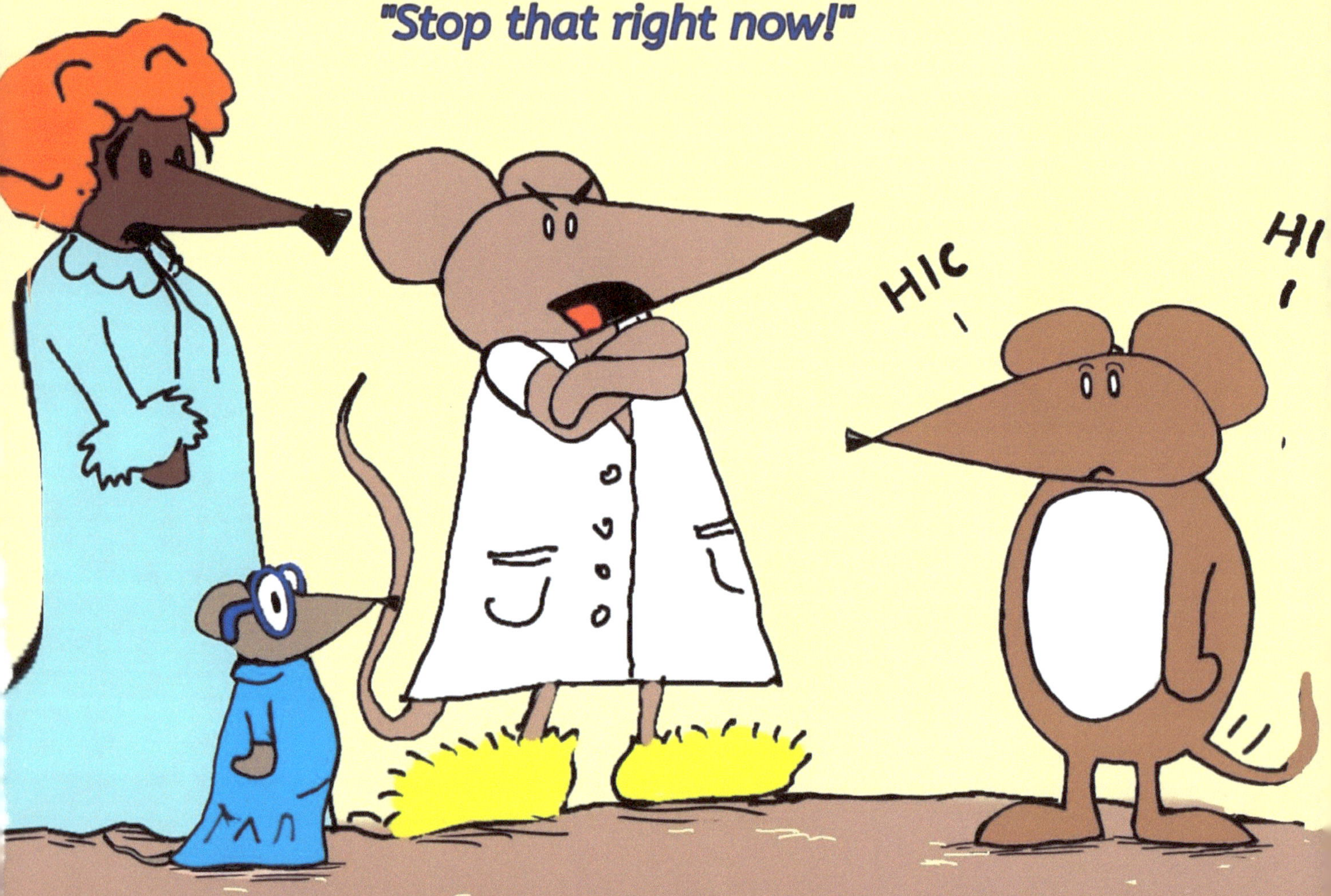

But Tommy hiccuped instead
because he didn't know how.

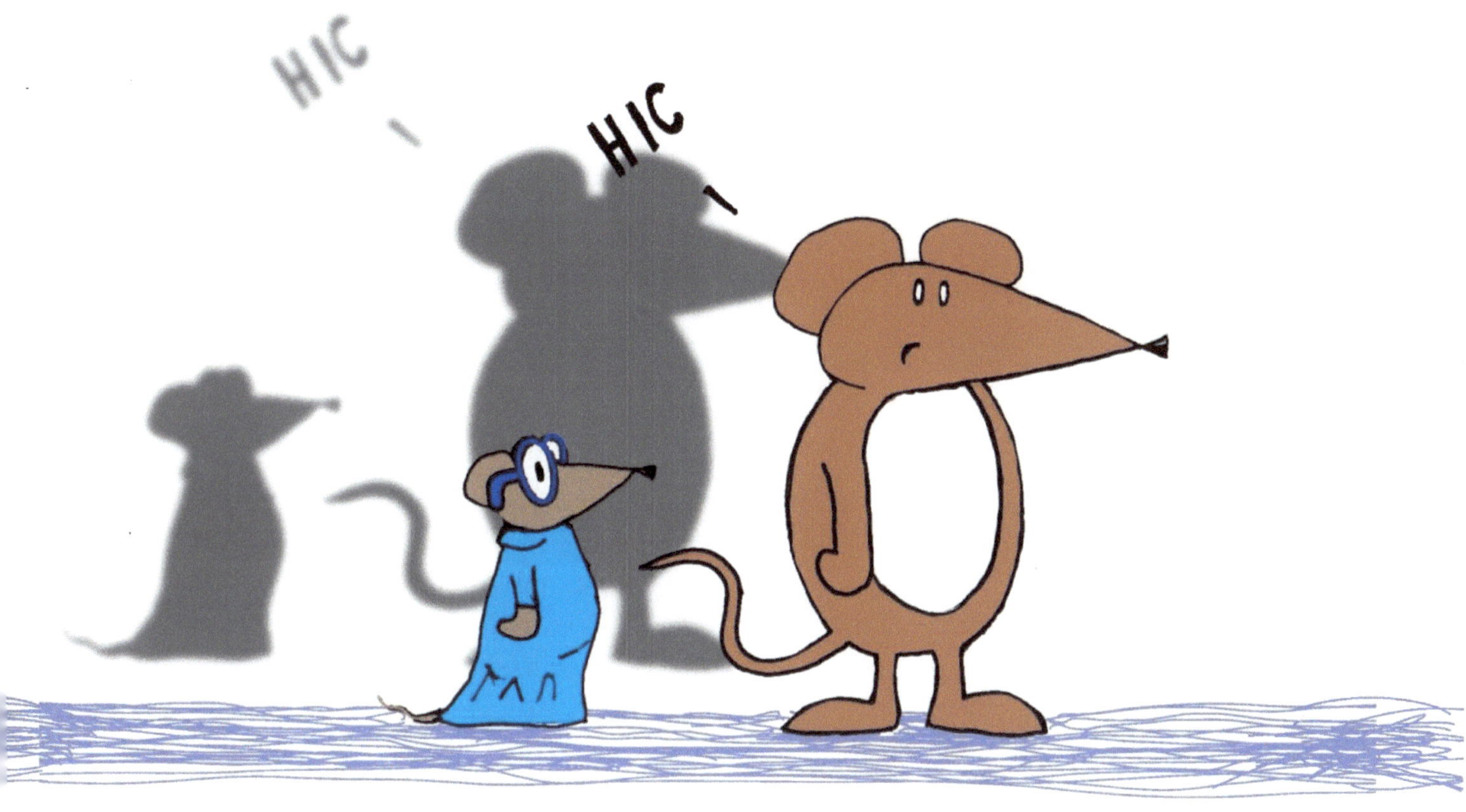

He waited and waited, but they only went HIC!

So he ran and asked everyone if they had a trick.

Ron was the first, he said "Put your face in this sack." Little brother Arthur made him take the sack back.

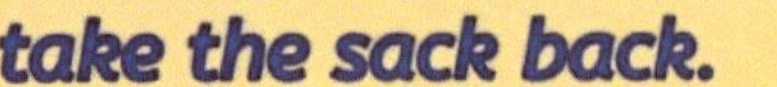
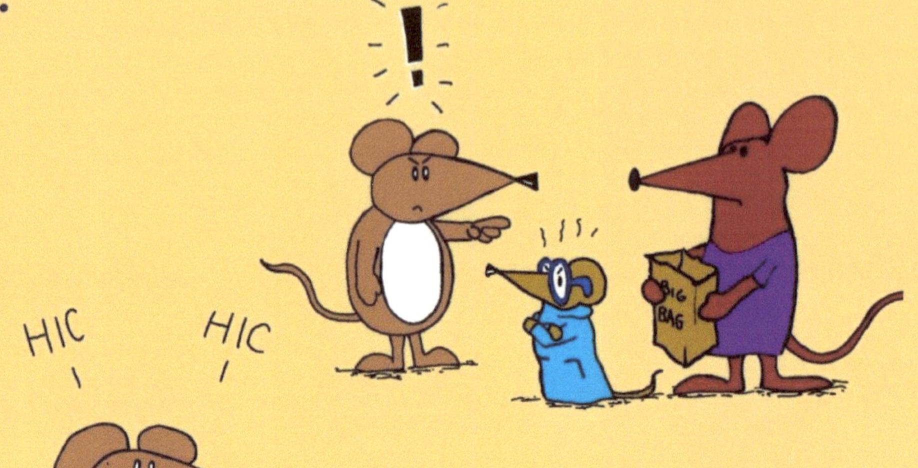

!
HIC
HIC
BIG
BAG

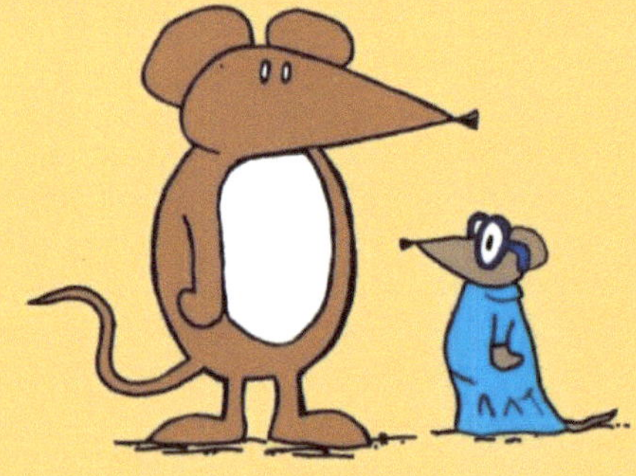

HIC

Sally, she tried to give him a scare! But no matter how much he shivered the hiccups stayed there.

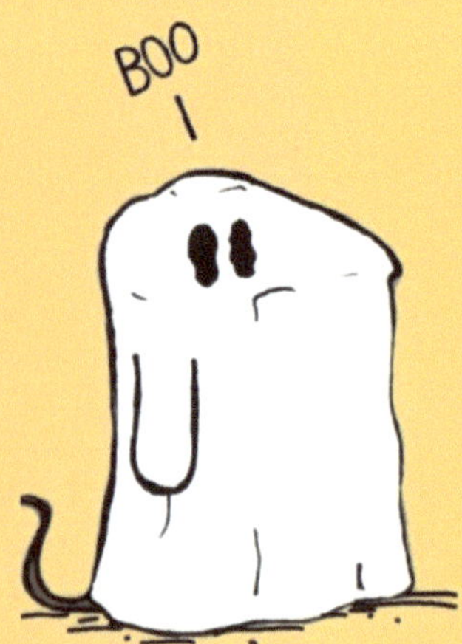

BOO

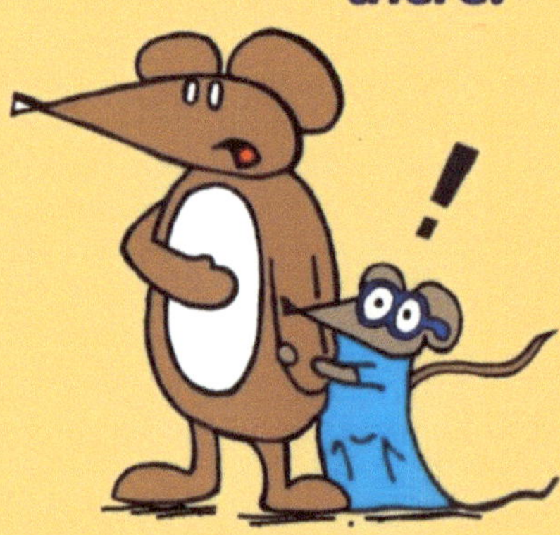

HIC
!

Ron had him drink from the wrong side of the
cup. He spilled it on Arthur on the very next
hiccup.

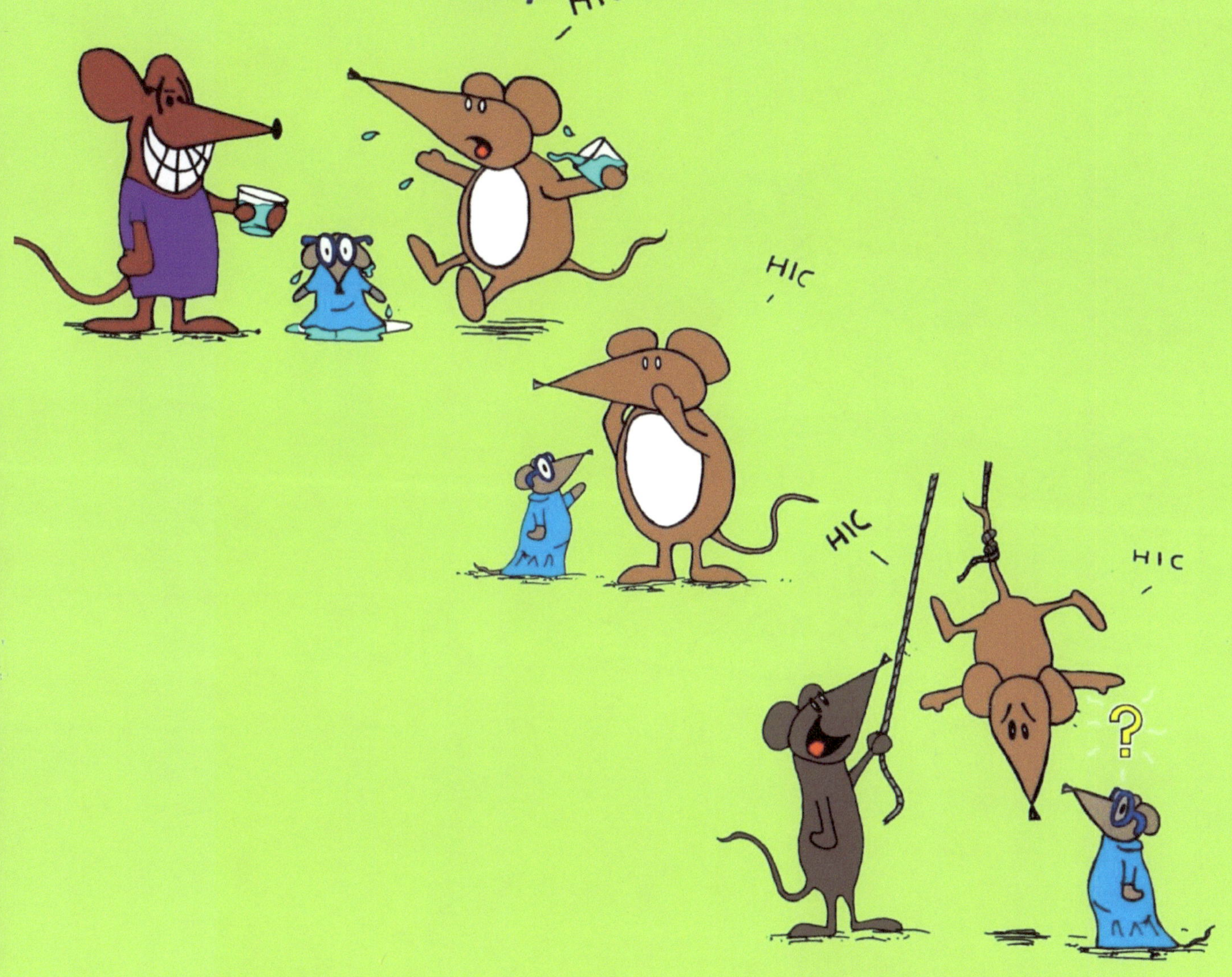

And then he tried hanging upside down by his tail.
Just like everything else, that was a fail.

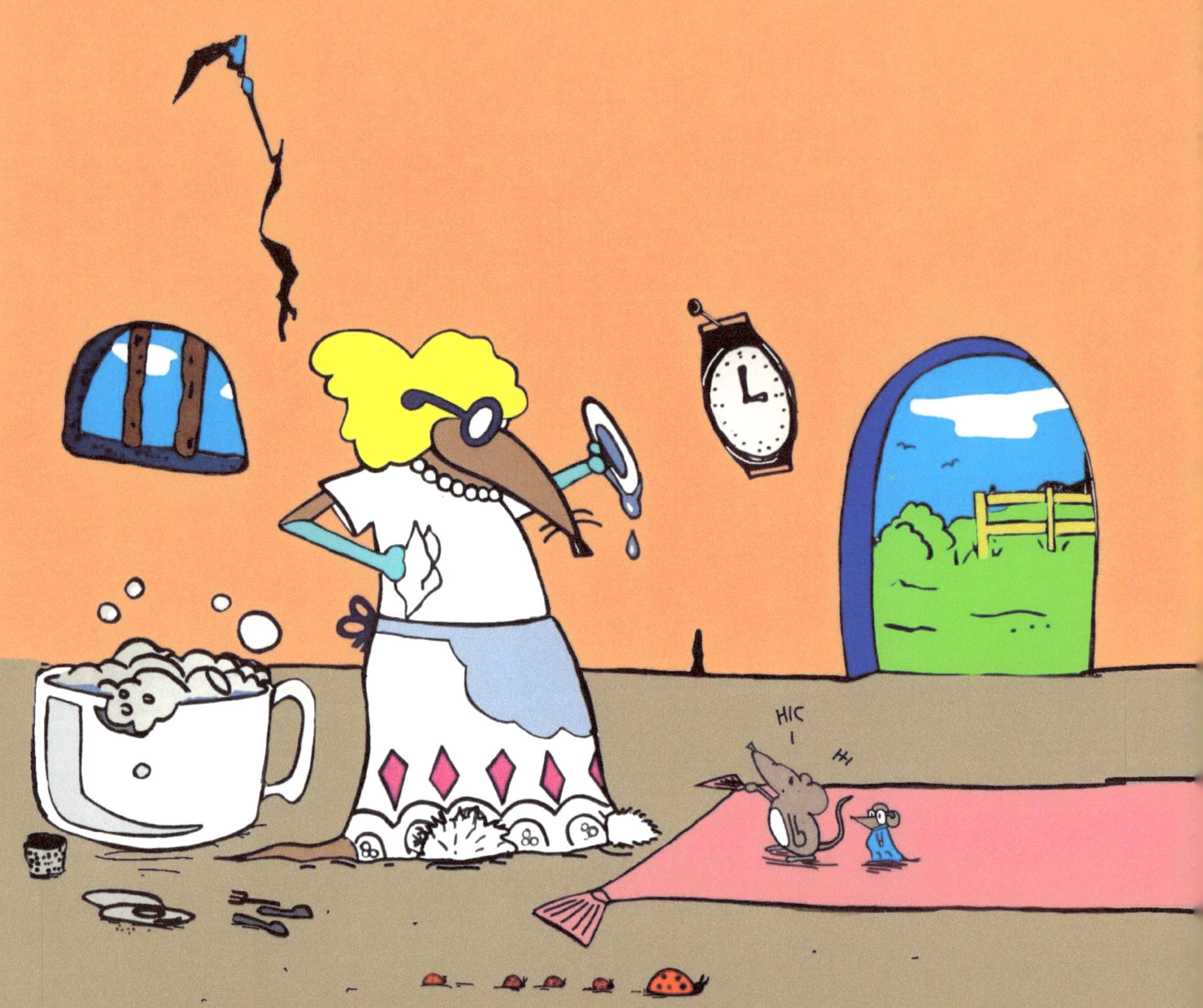

"Grandma, how do I stop these hiccups of mine?"

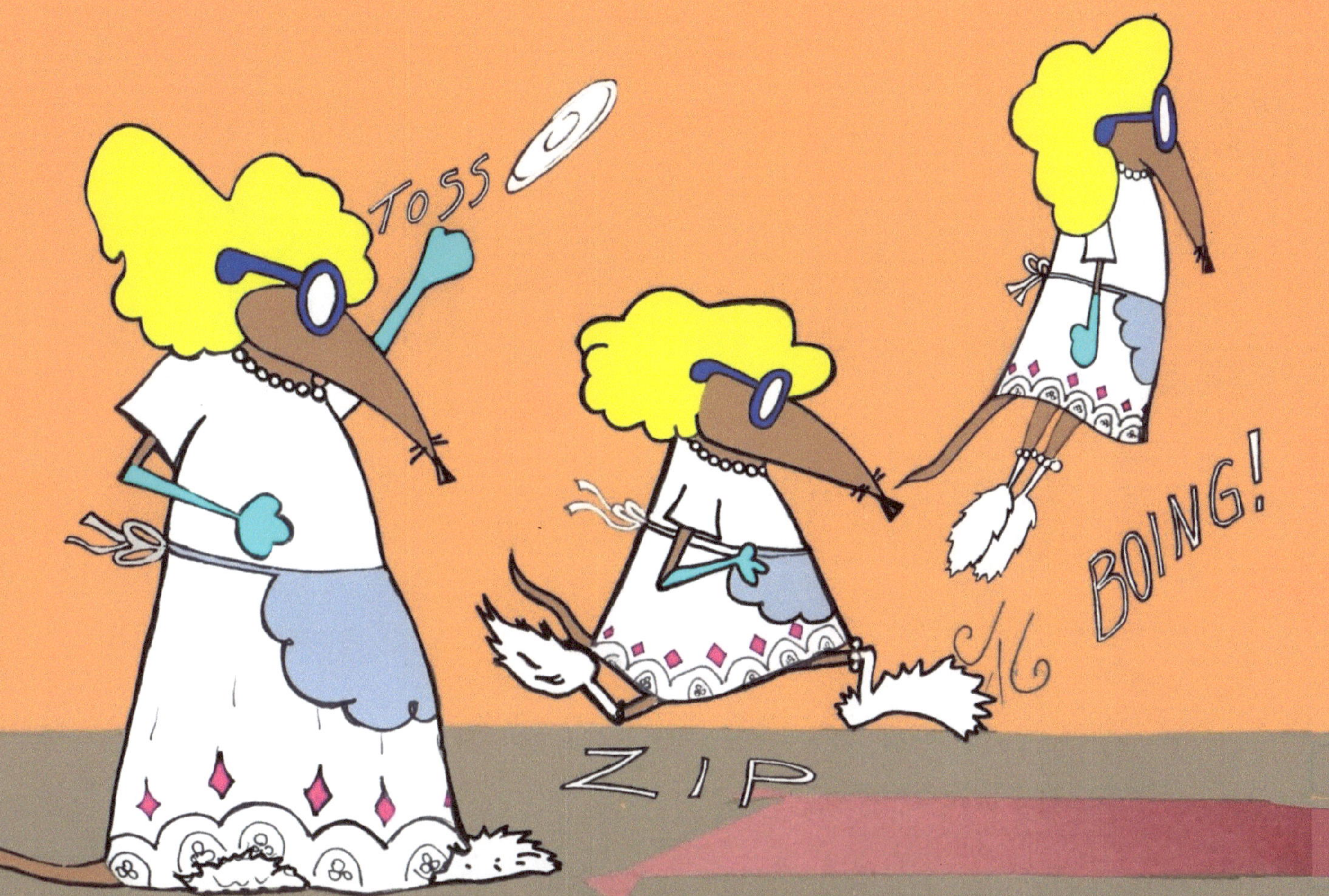

"I know exactly what to do!" Said Grandma.
TOSS
ZIP
BOING!
"This works every time!"

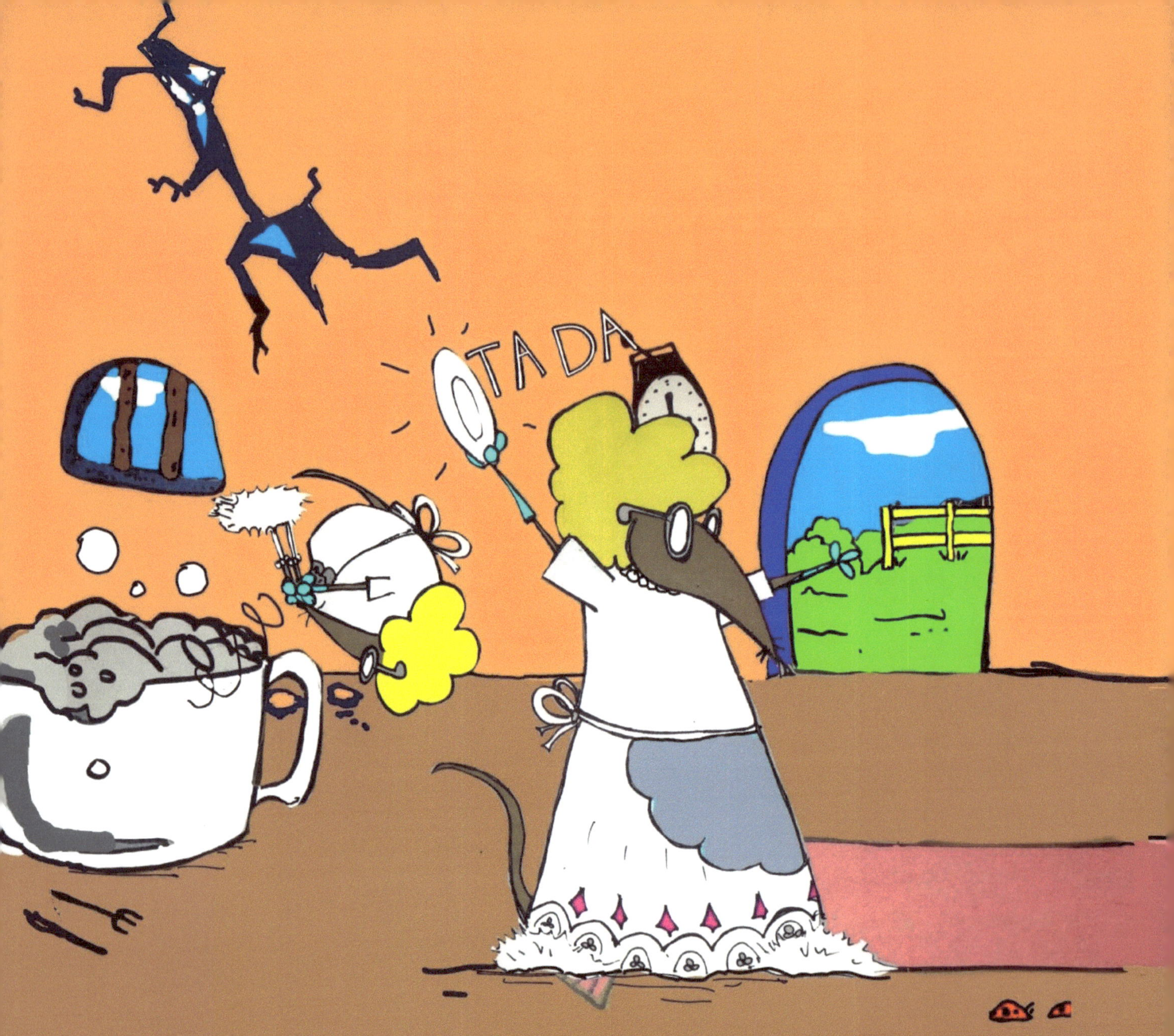

She zipped and she flipped and flew in the air!

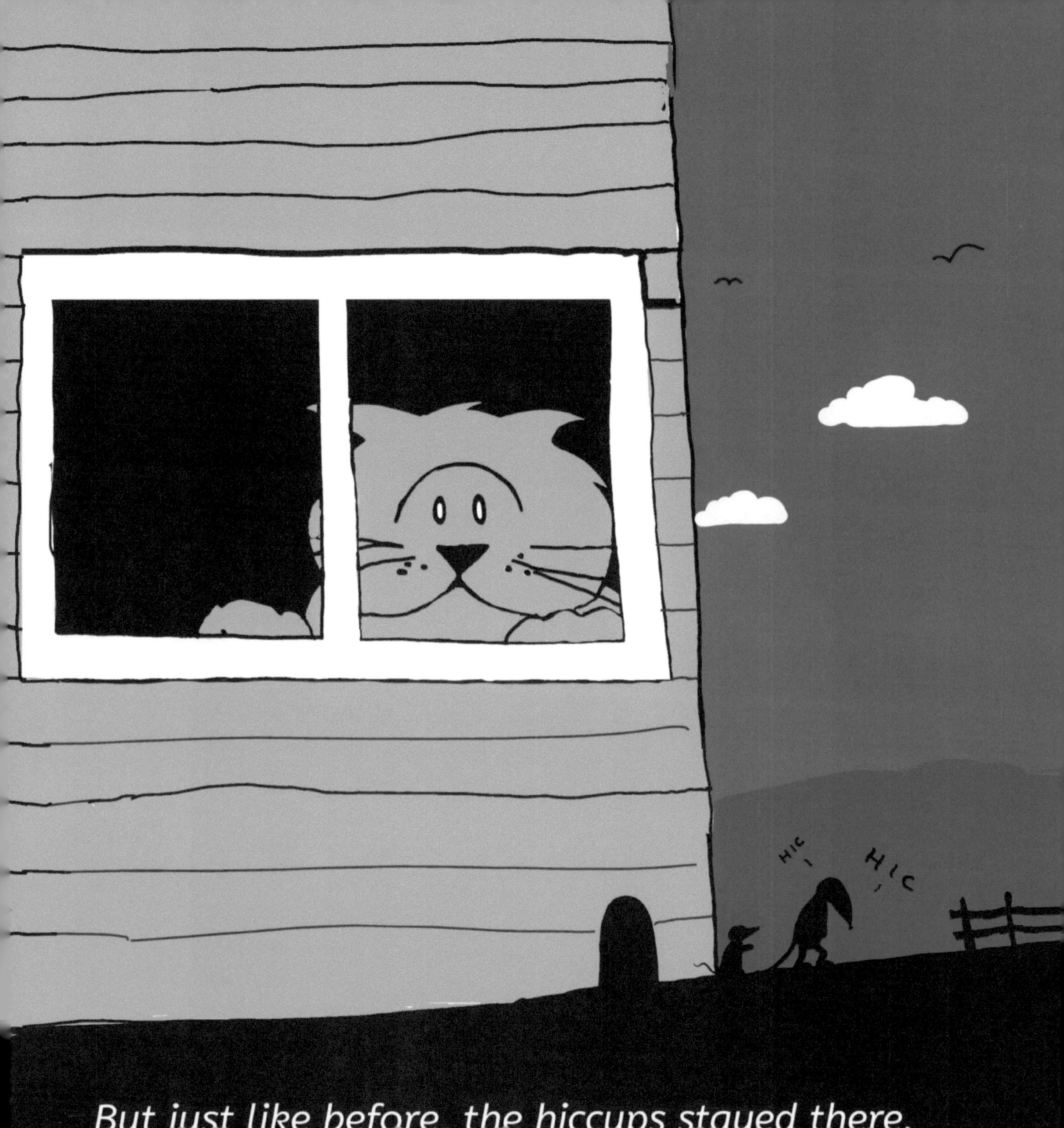

But just like before, the hiccups stayed there.

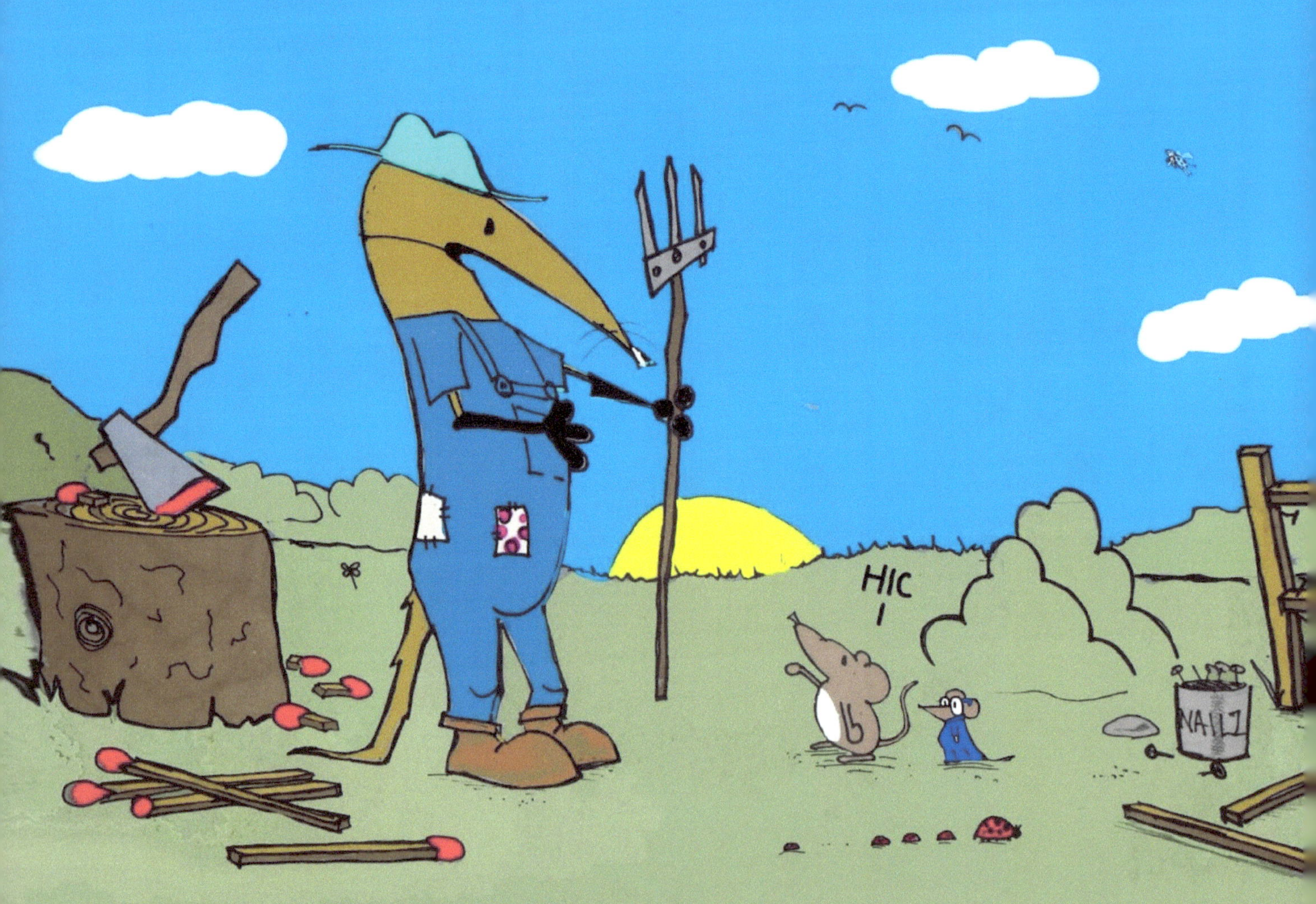

"Oh Grandpa please I have the hiccups bad,

can I get the cure from you?"

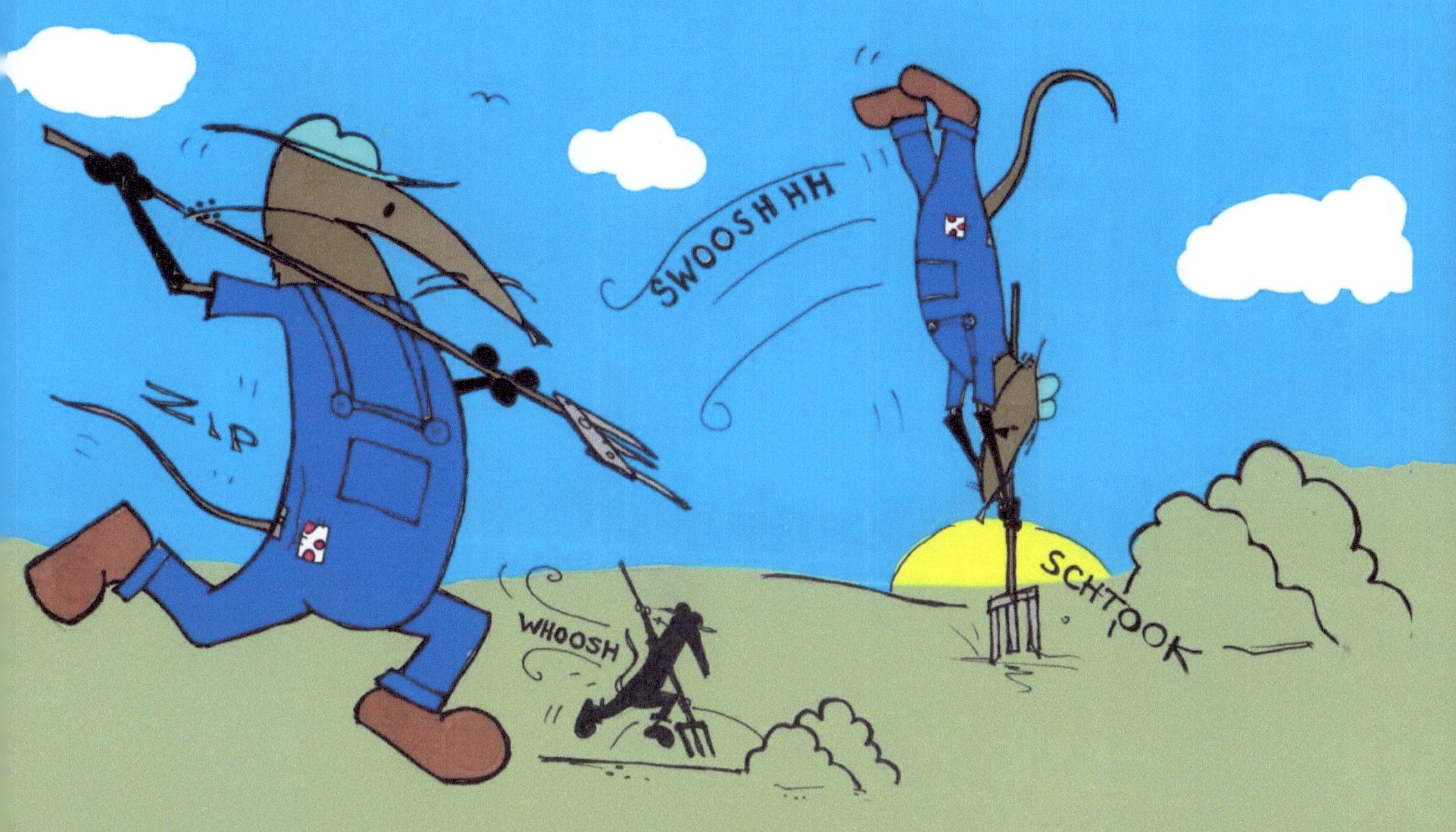

Grampa said,"Take a step back lad.

I know exactly what to do!"

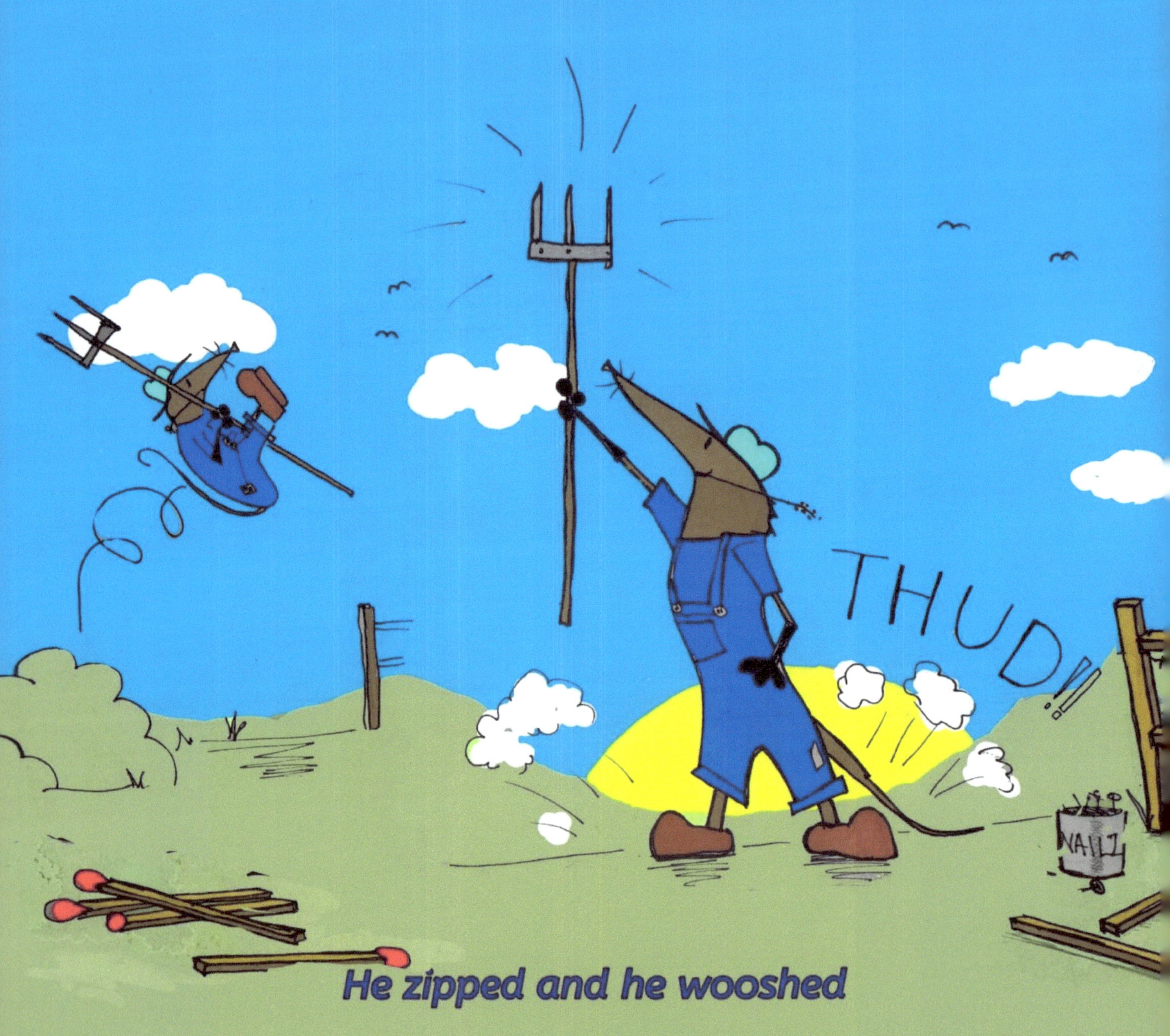

He zipped and he wooshed

and landed quite hard!

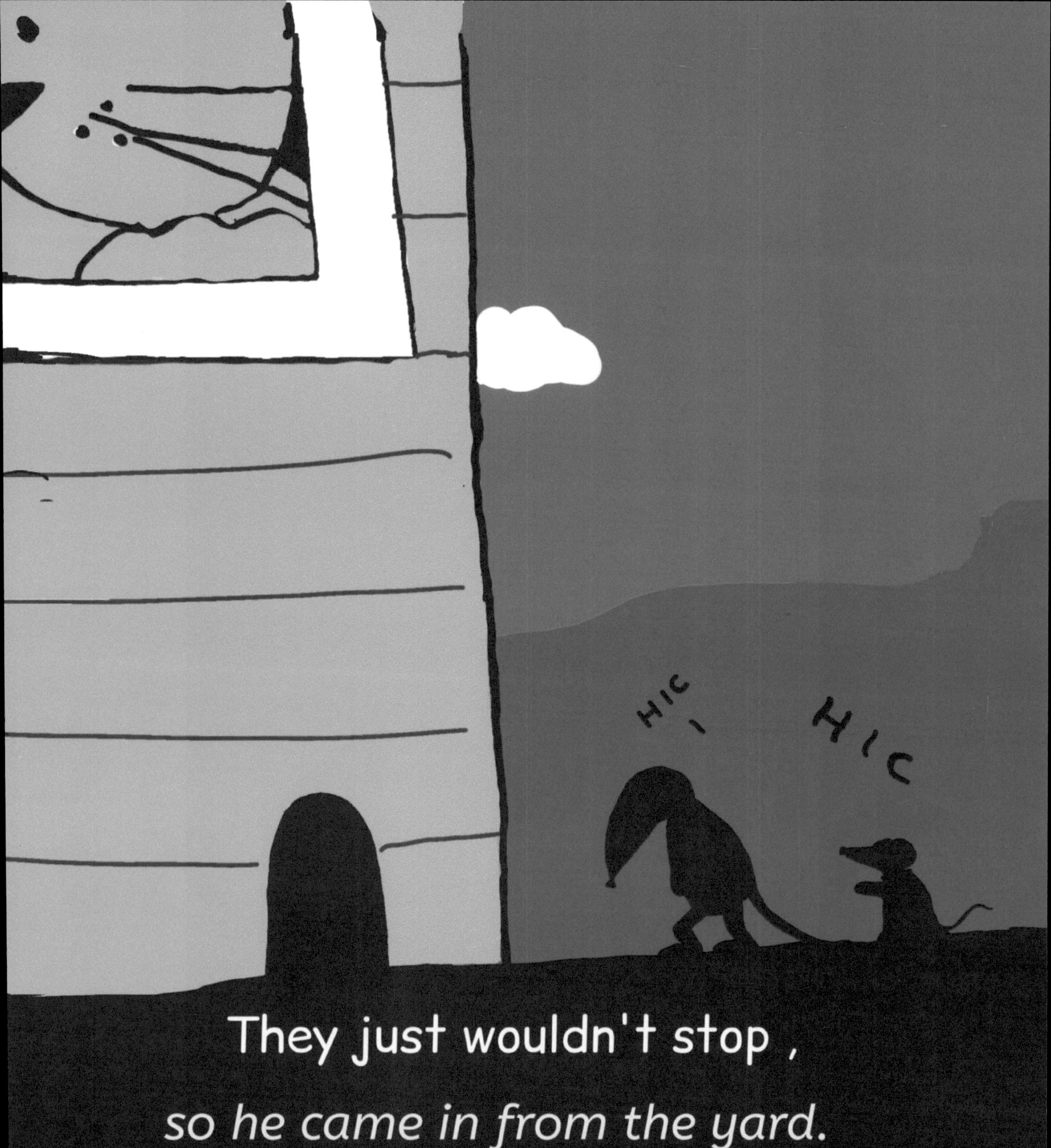

They just wouldn't stop ,
so he came in from the yard.

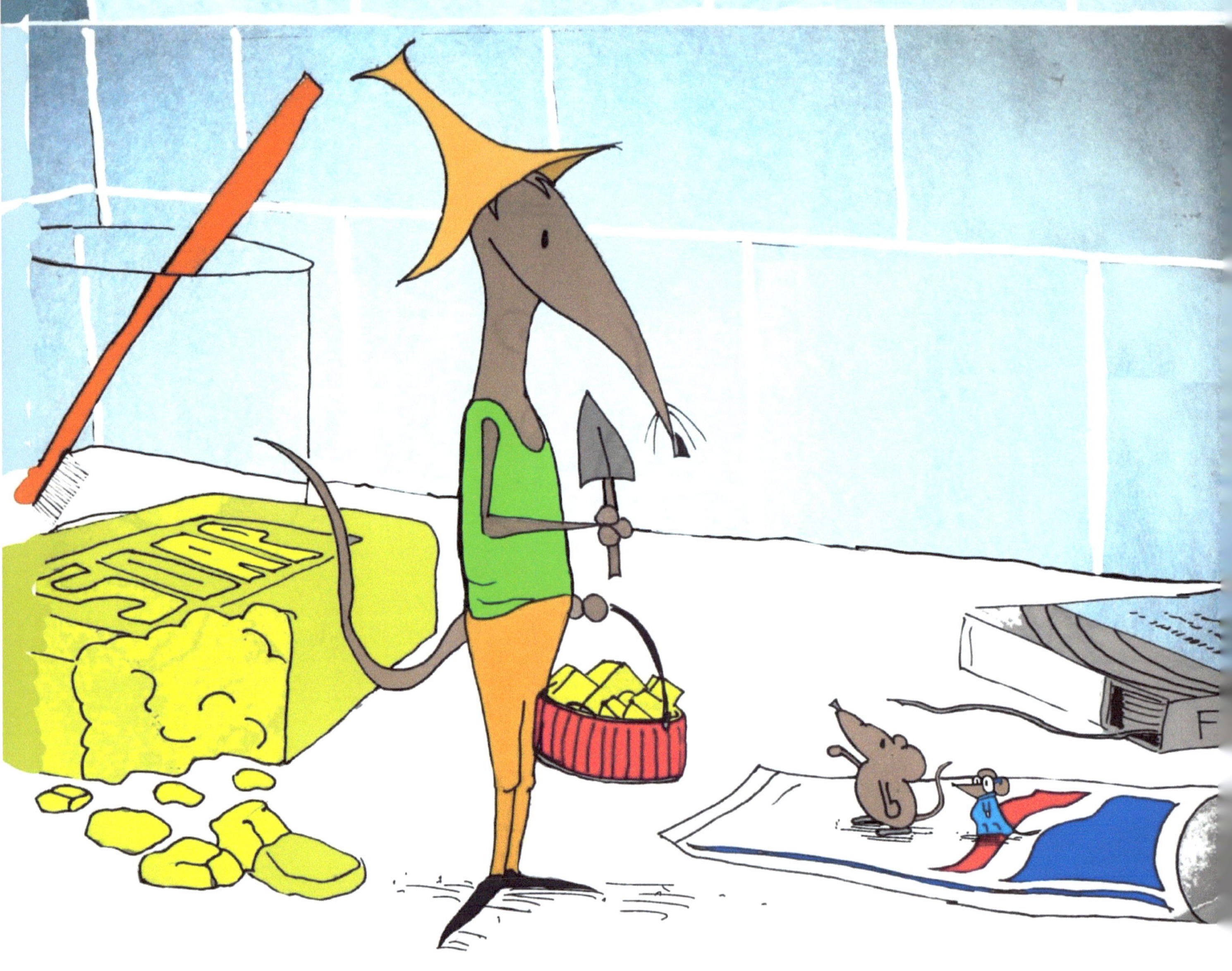

"Please help me Uncle Ray,

I've hiccuped all day!"

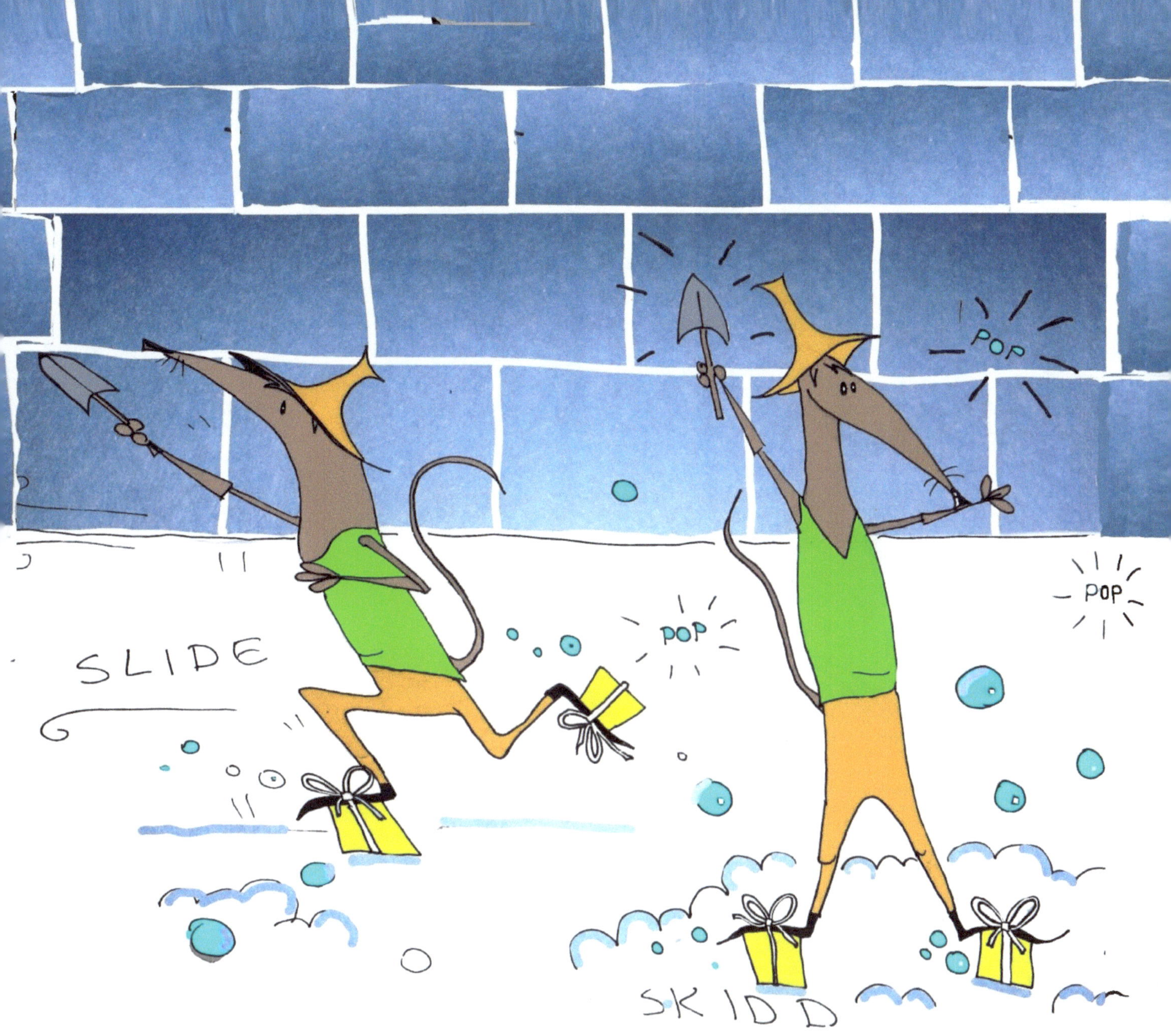

"A quick scrub and some suds makes it all go away!"

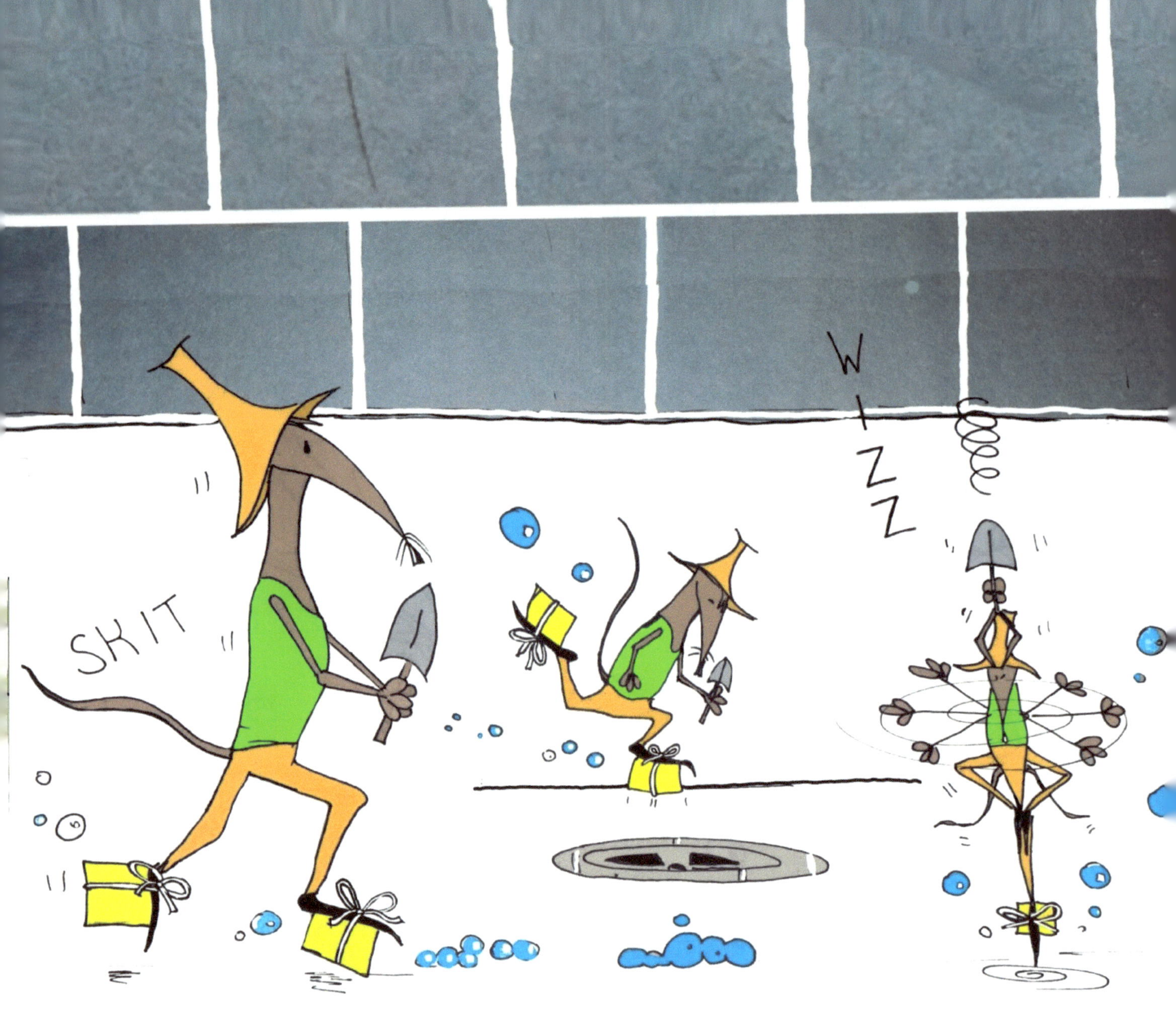

So he skated and twirled and made a quick stop!

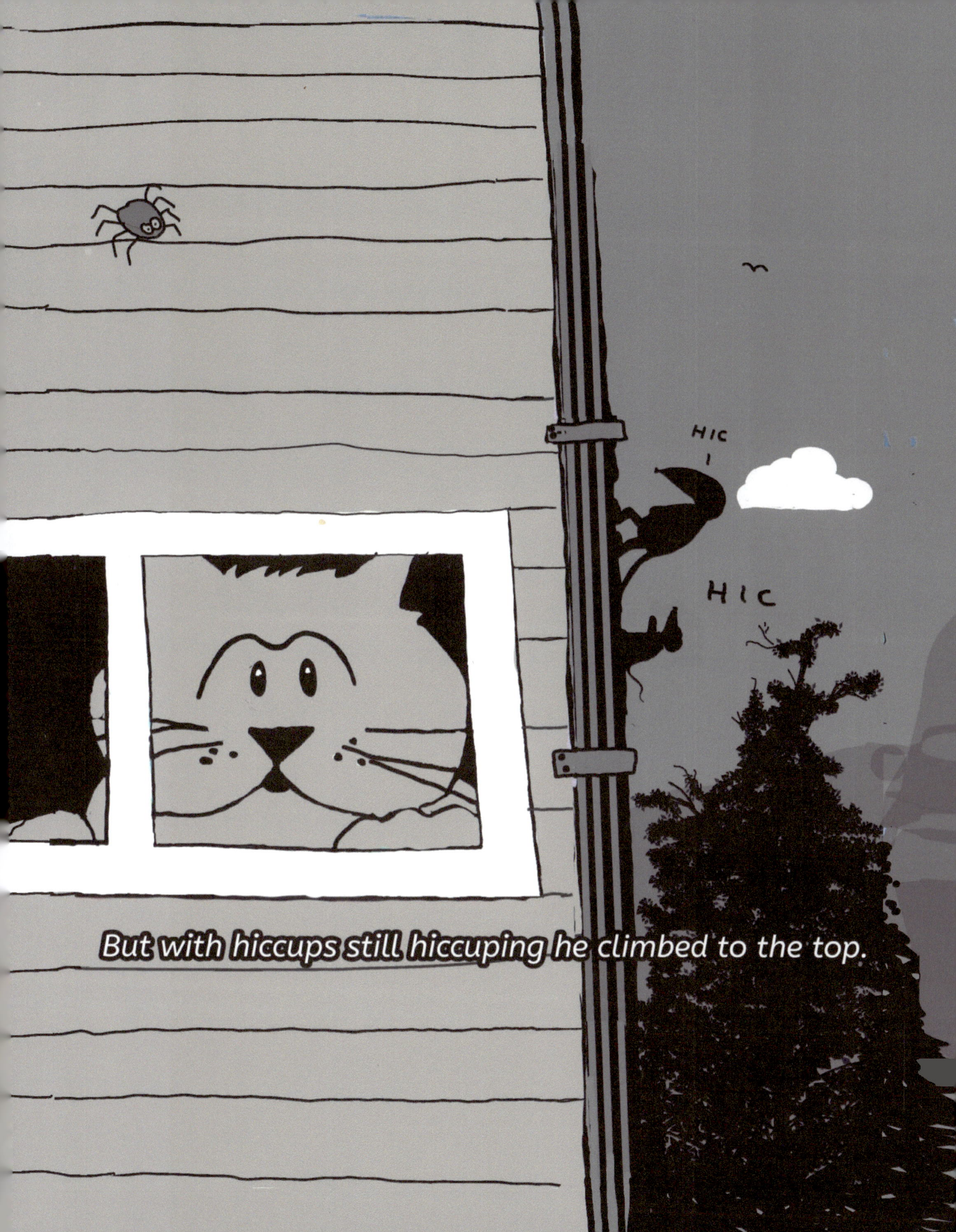

But with hiccups still hiccuping he climbed to the top.

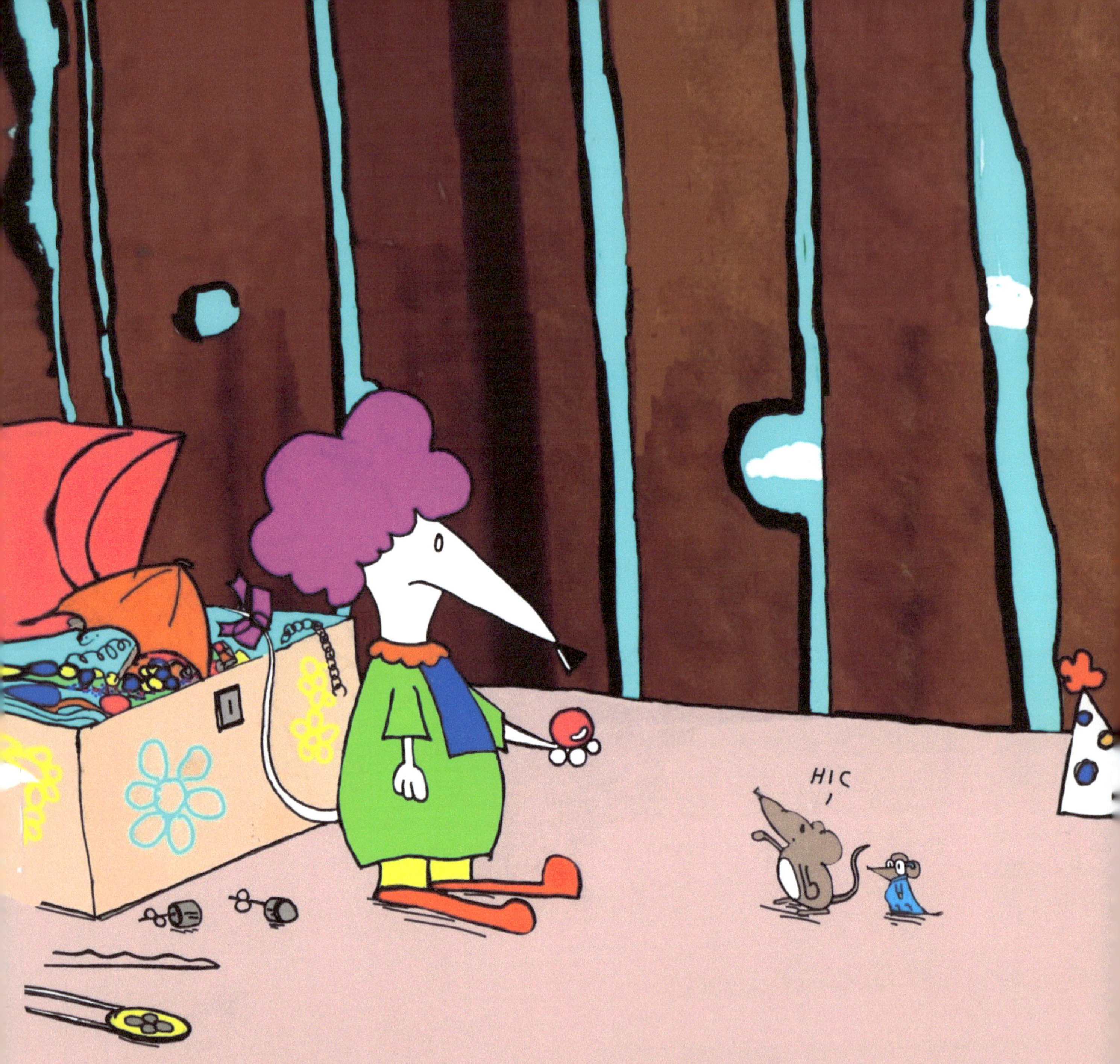

Aunt Betty, oh please, I've asked everyone else!

I can't stop these hiccups all by myself!

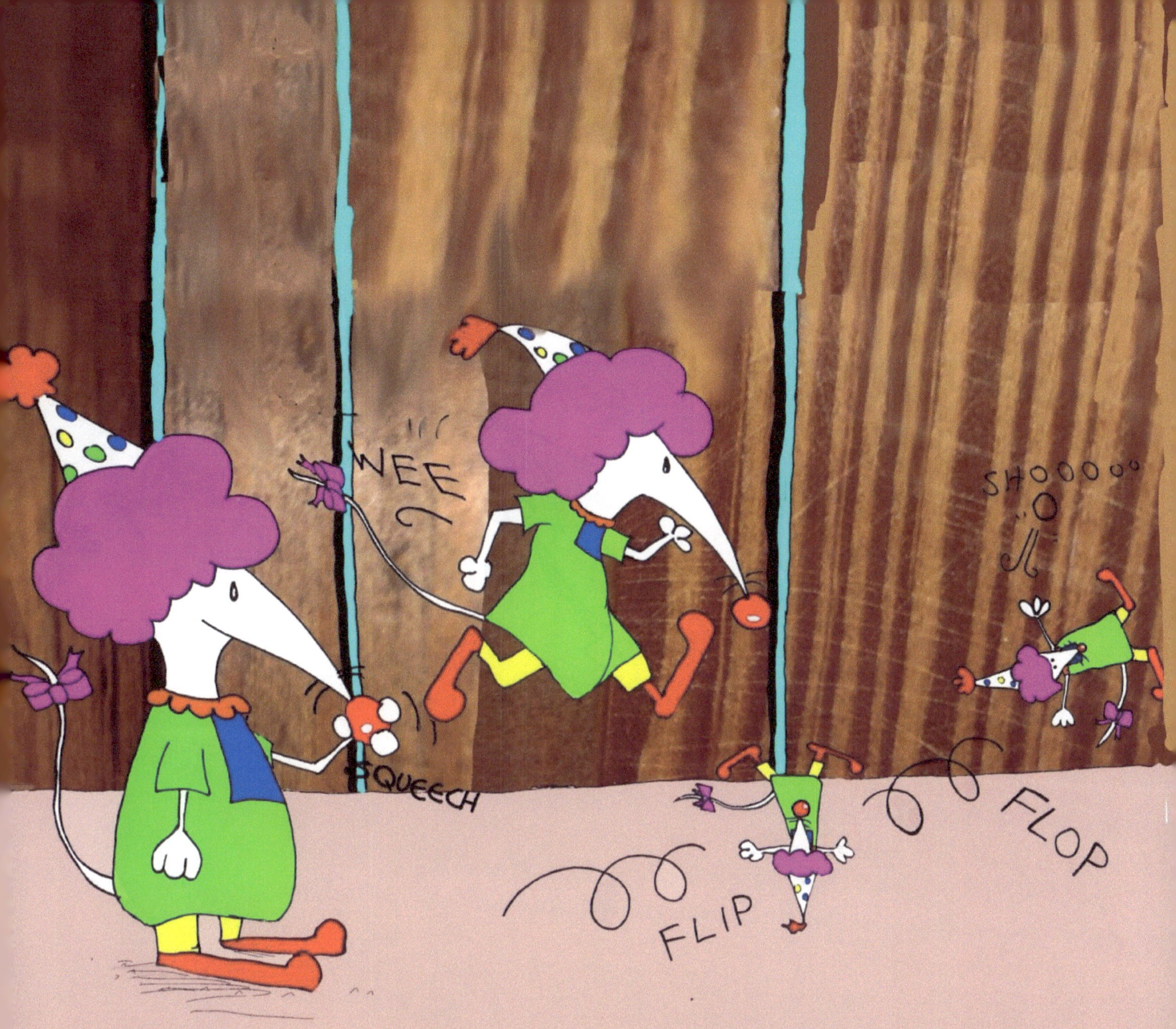

I can show you the way I did as a girl!

Then she flipped and she flopped

and she did a big twirl.

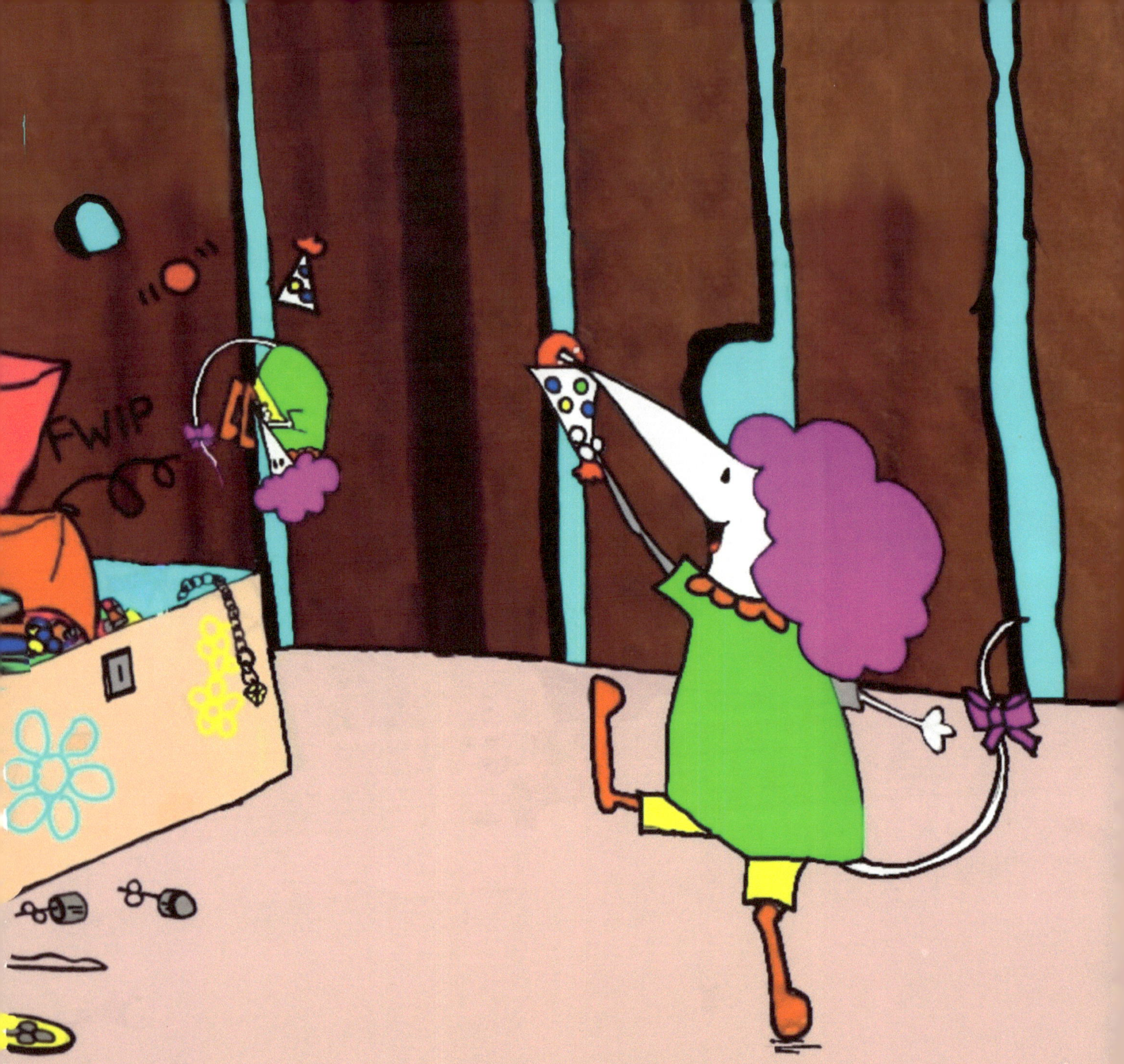

And when she was done
she caught her nose in her hat!

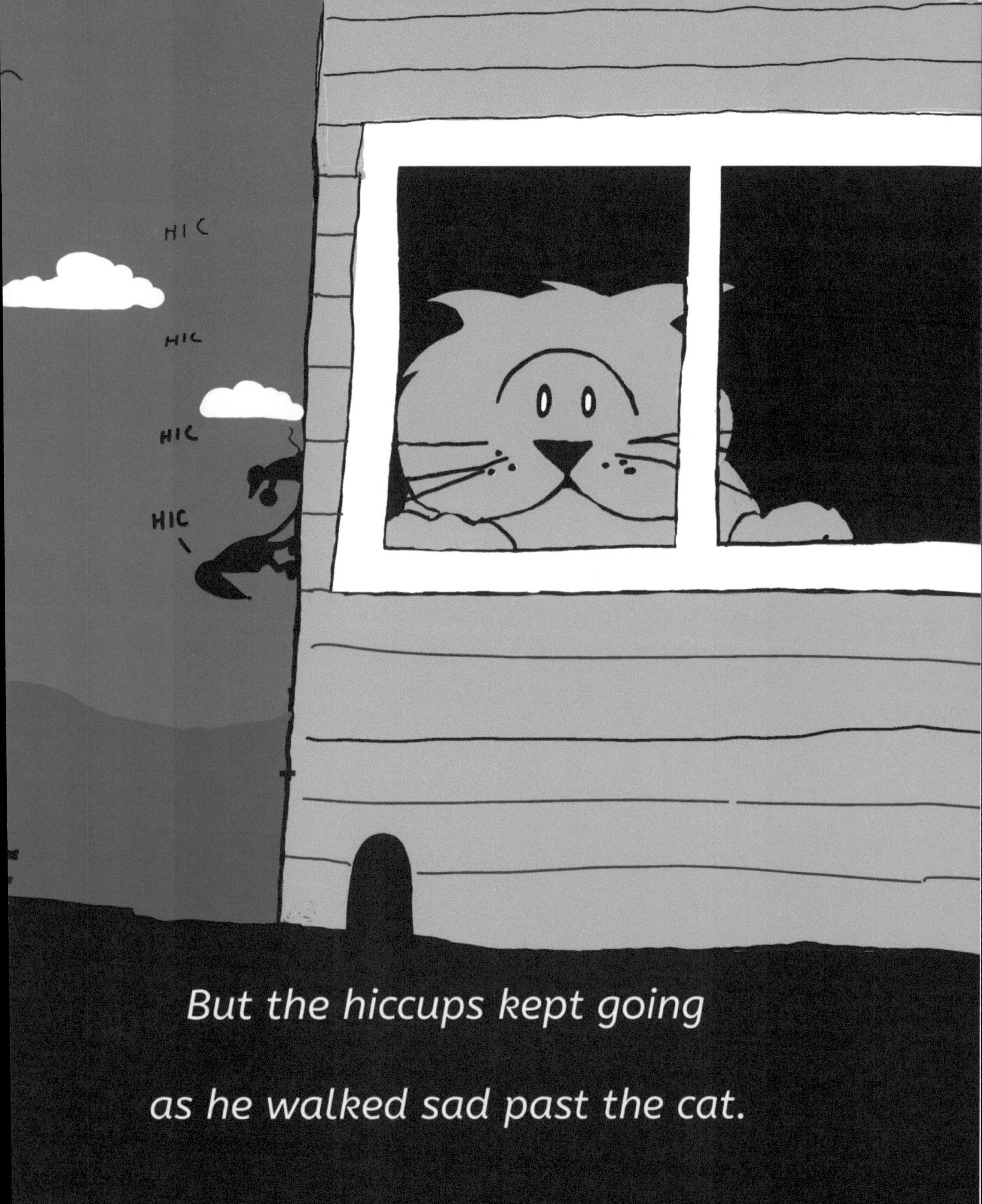

But the hiccups kept going

as he walked sad past the cat.

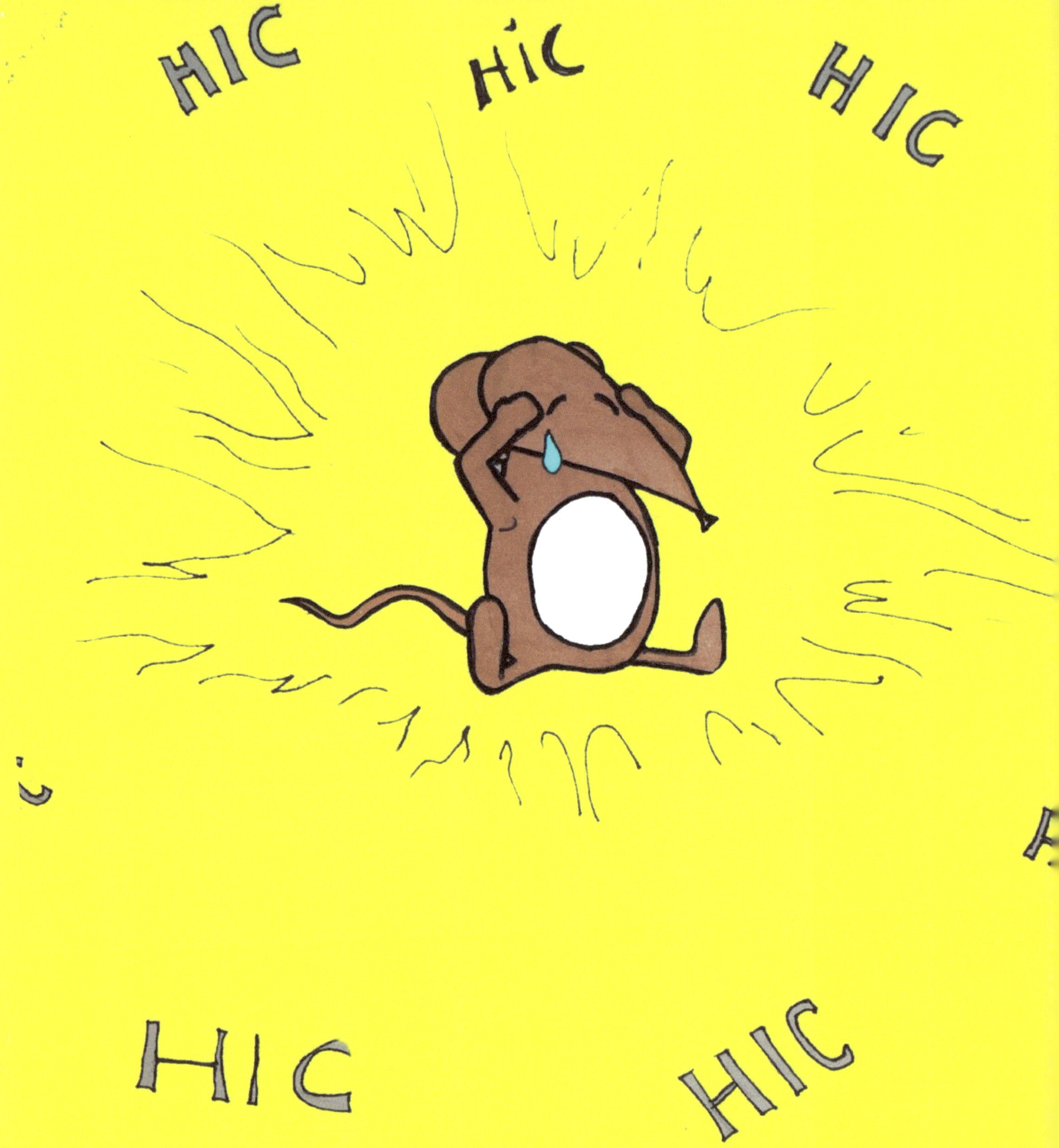

HIC
HIC
HIC
HIC
HIC
HIC

Little Arthur spoke up and told him...

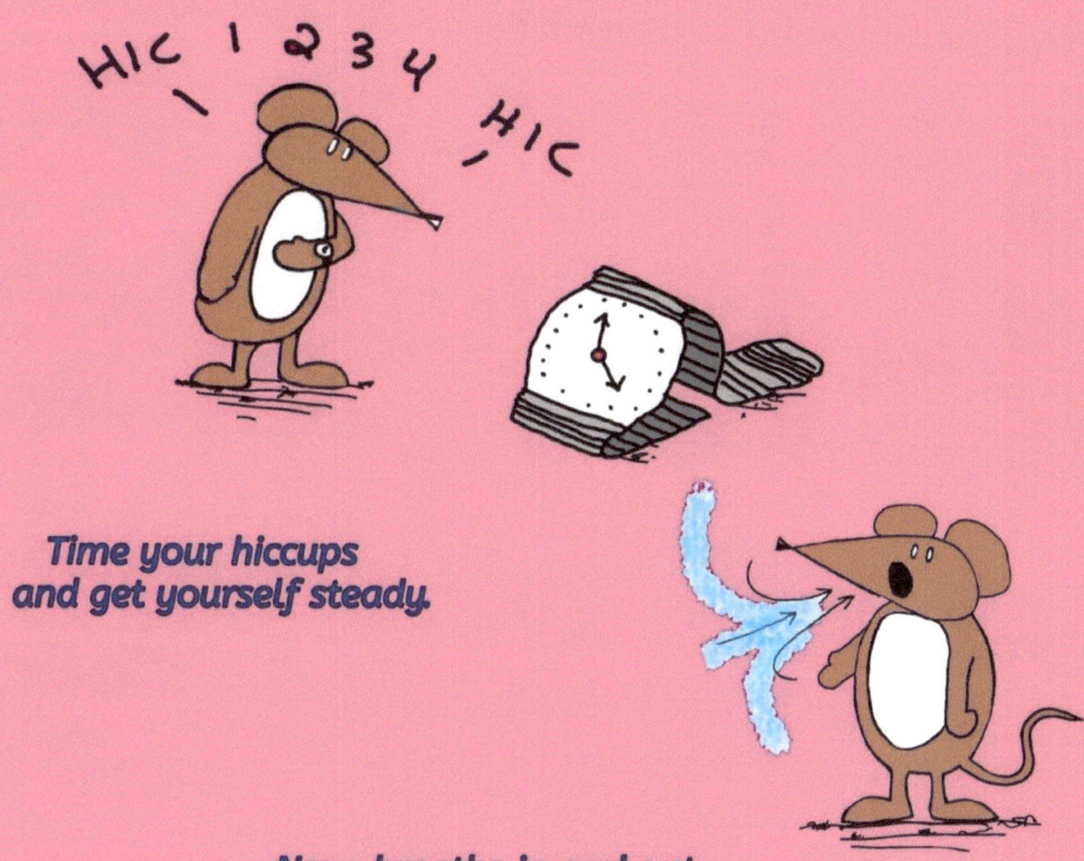

**Time your hiccups
and get yourself steady.**

**Now, breathe in and out
really deep and get ready!**

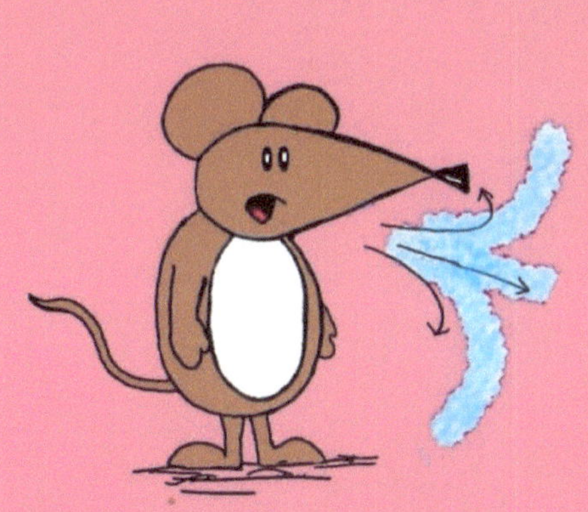

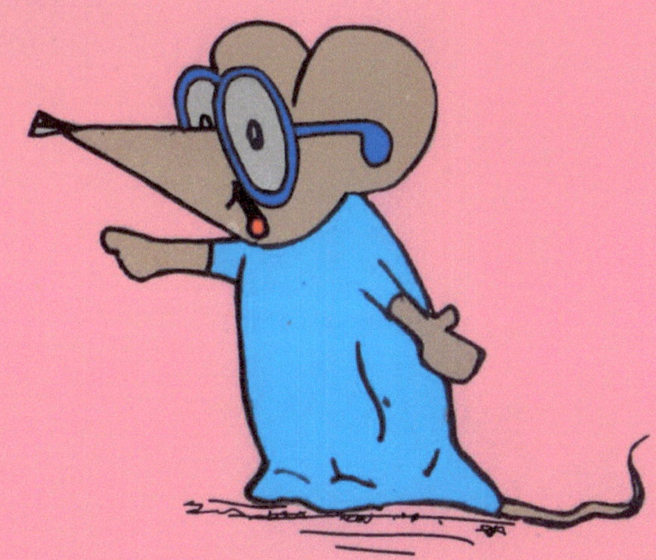

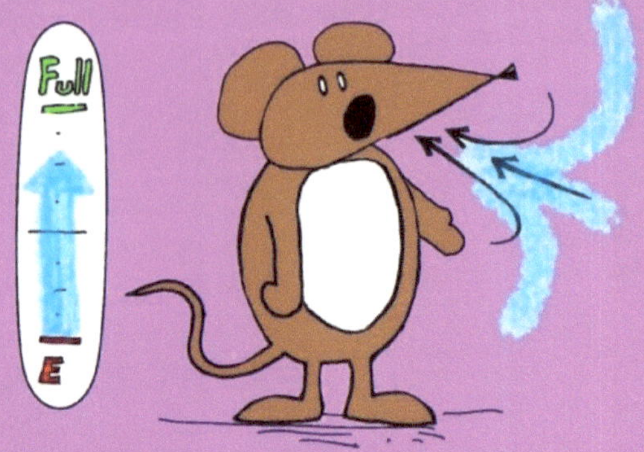

As soon as your hiccup is gone take a super deep breath, fill your lungs ALL THE WAY! Don't worry you won't have to hold it all day.

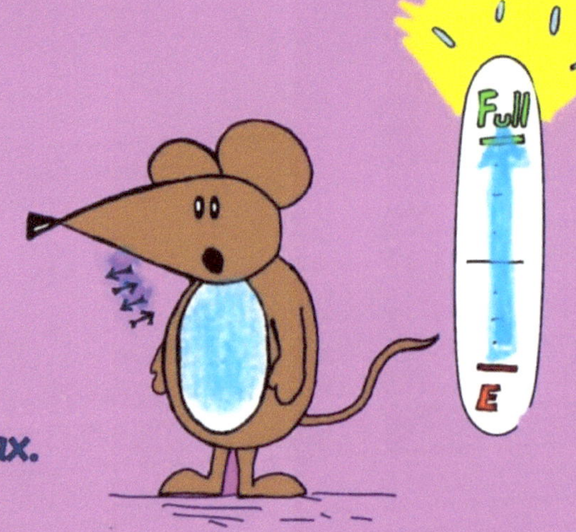

Now don't close your mouth,
there's no going back.
Just breathe tiny in an out
and keep your lungs packed and relax.

There should be no next hiccup,
and count to be sure we are there.
Be gentle and slowly
let out let out all the air.

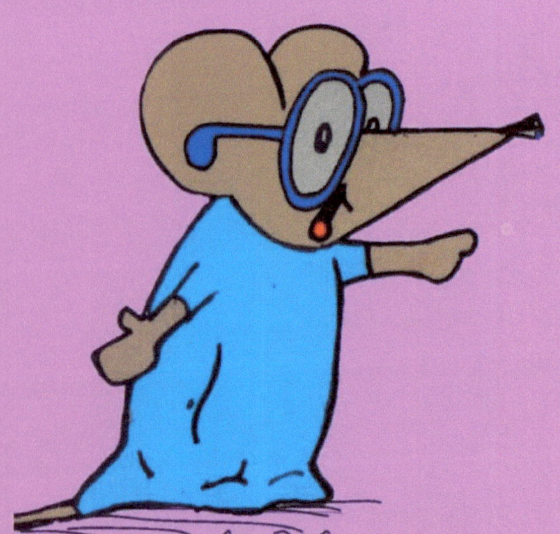

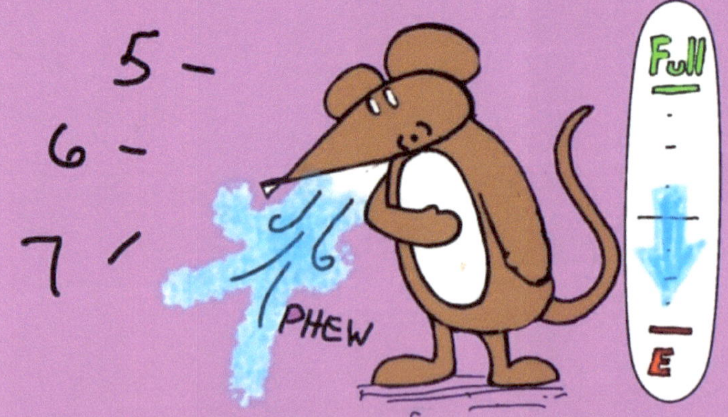

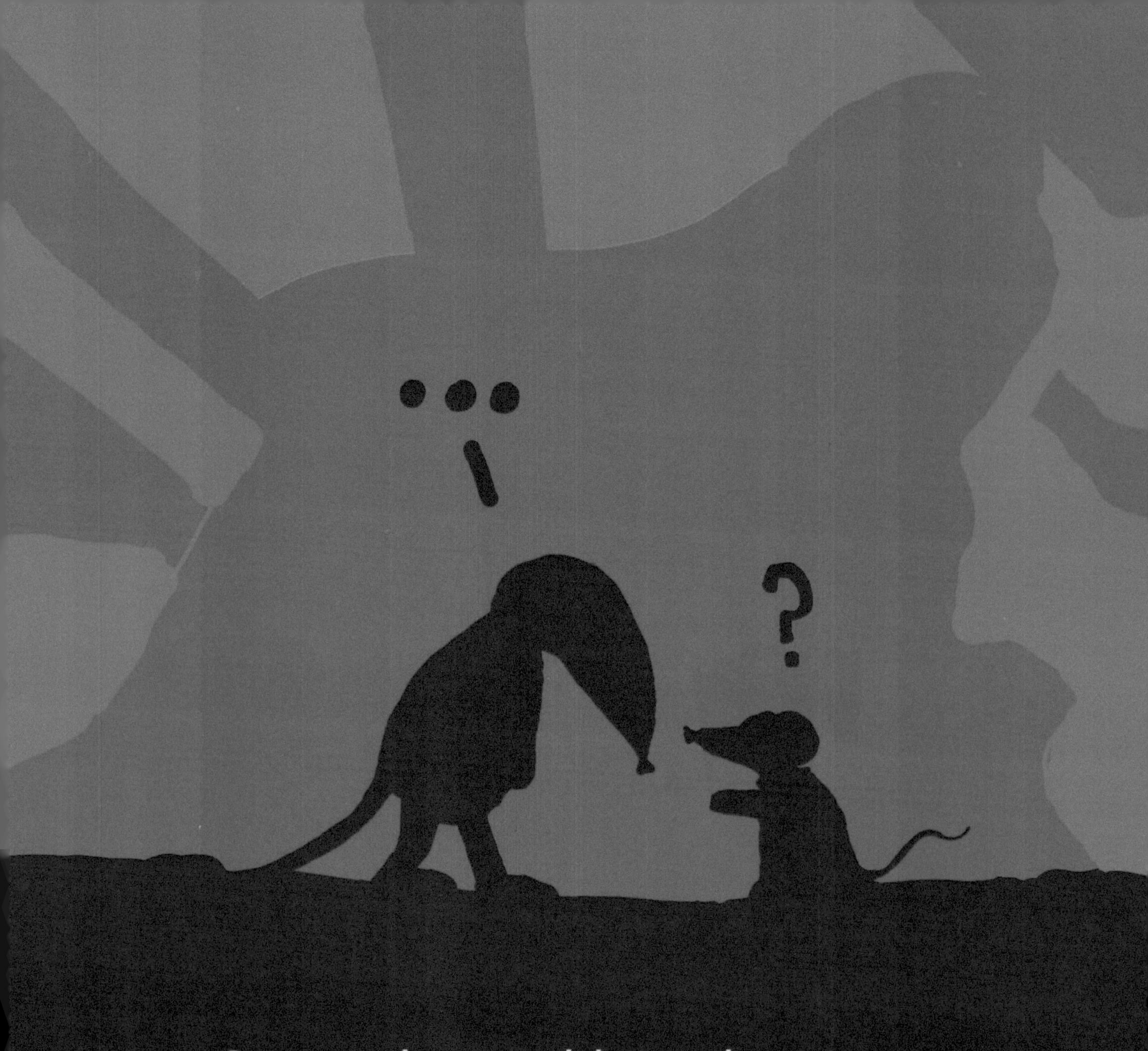

Stay calm and breathe easy,
a quick breath brings them back.
If they do, try again
and remember, RELAX

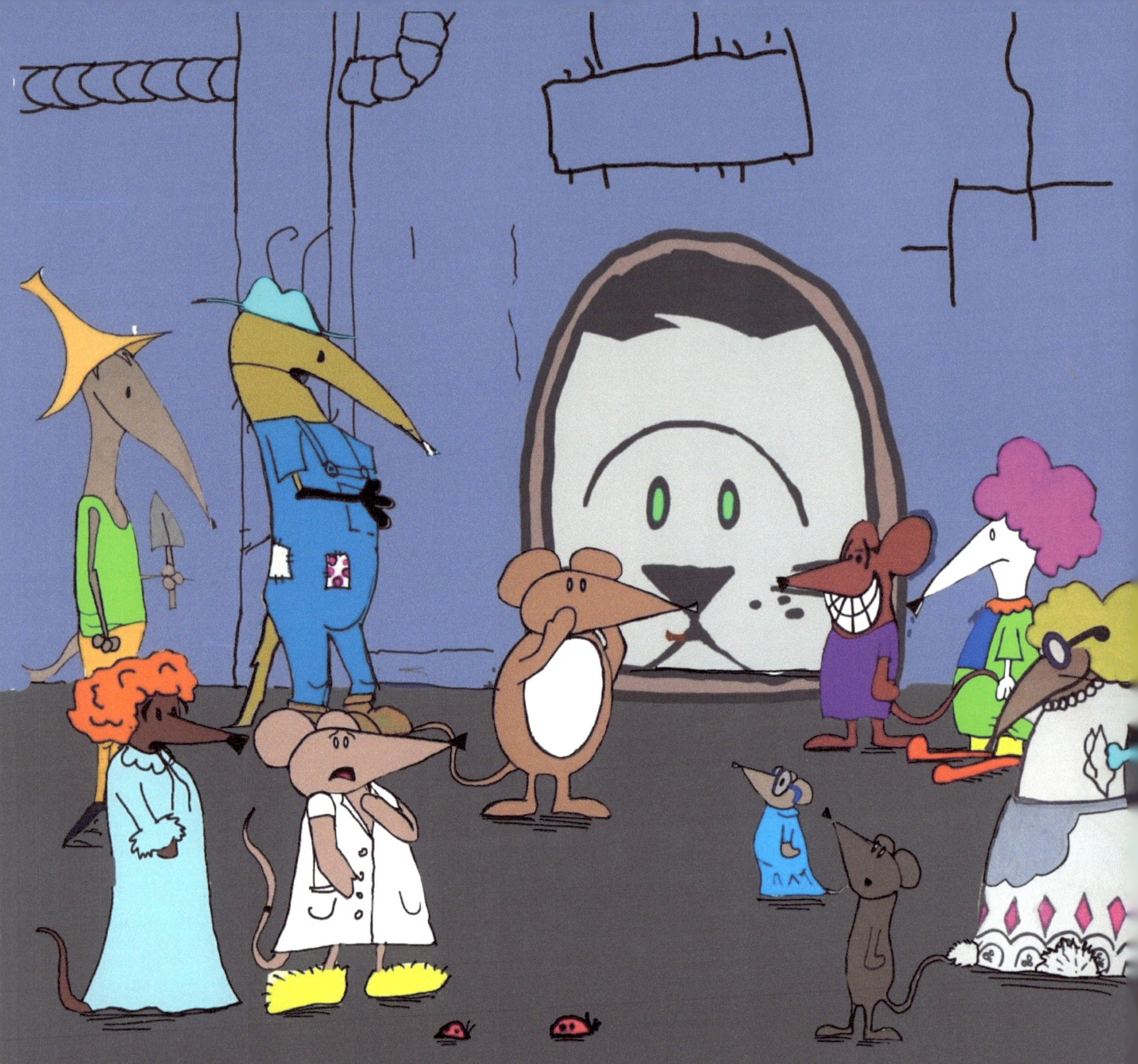
Everyone listened.
"Had they stopped?"
They all gasped.

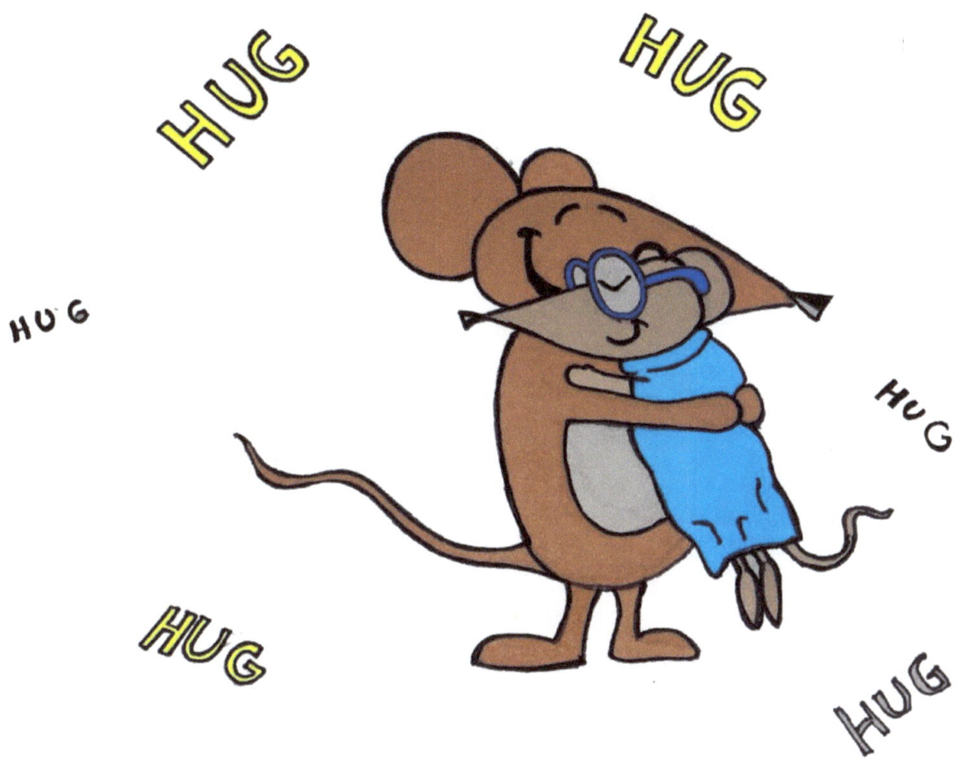

THE HORRIBLE HICCUPS HAD HALTED AT LAST!

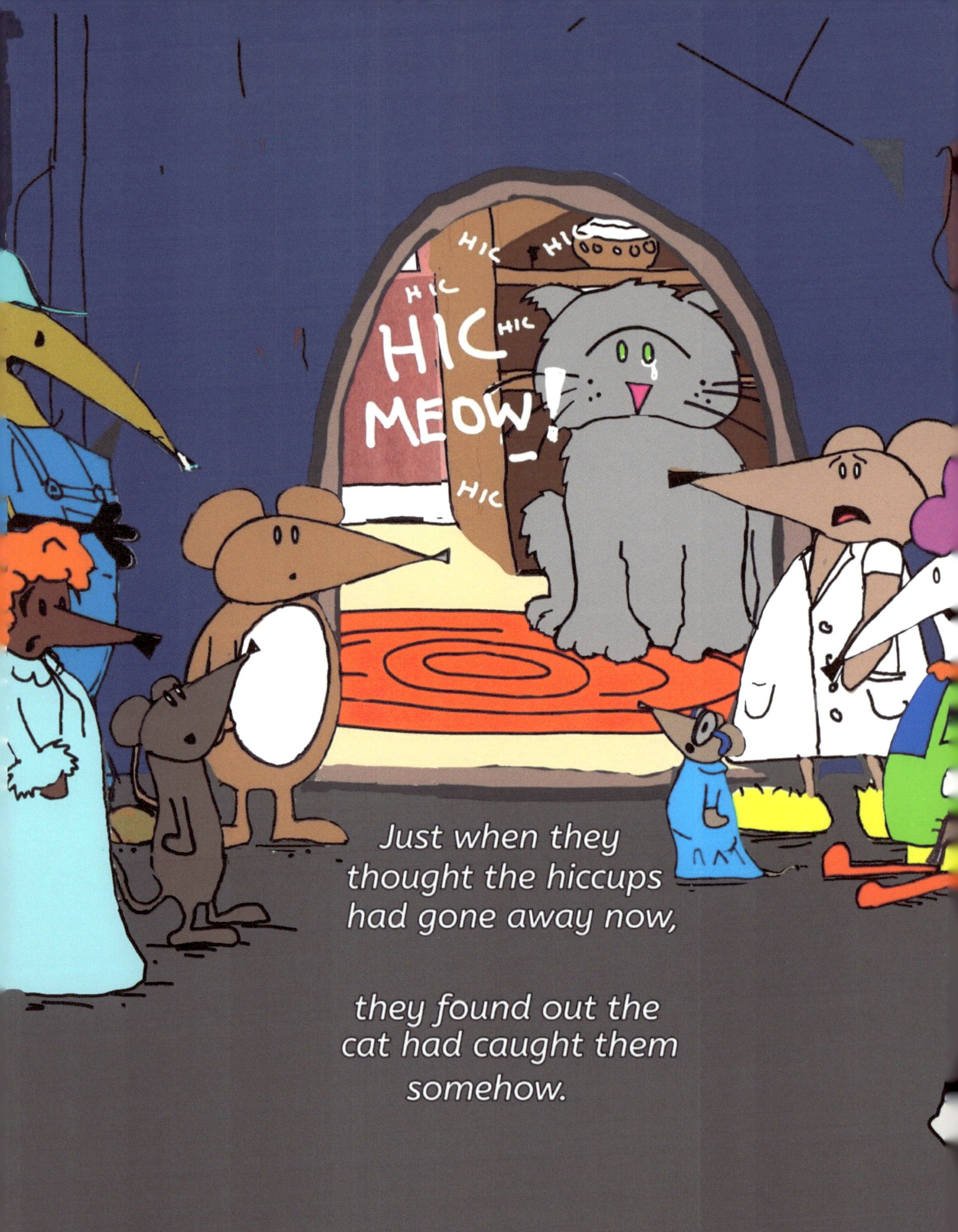

Just when they thought the hiccups had gone away now,

they found out the cat had caught them somehow.

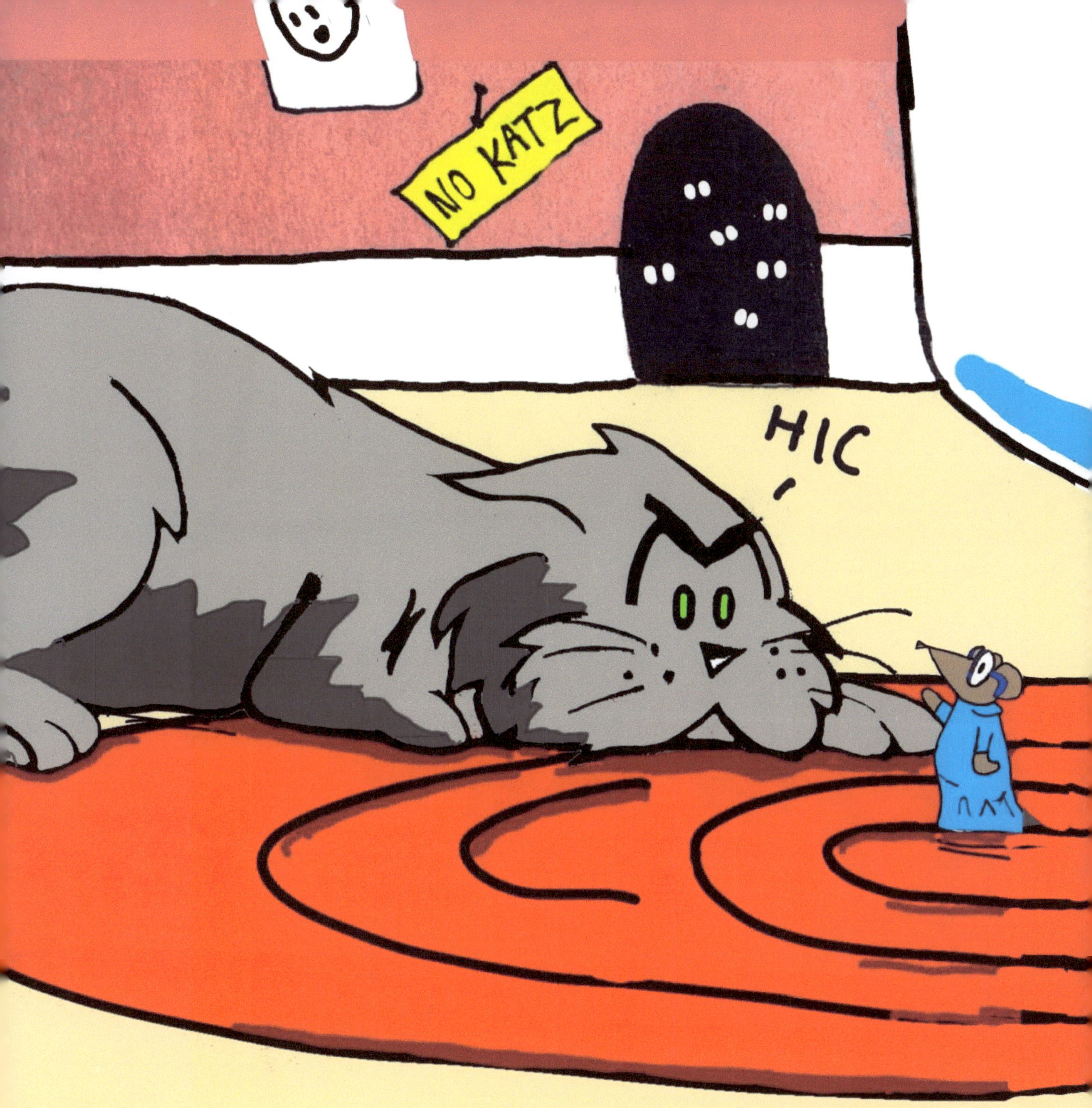

Arthur dashed out as brave as could be!
He told the big kitty his steps 1 2 3!

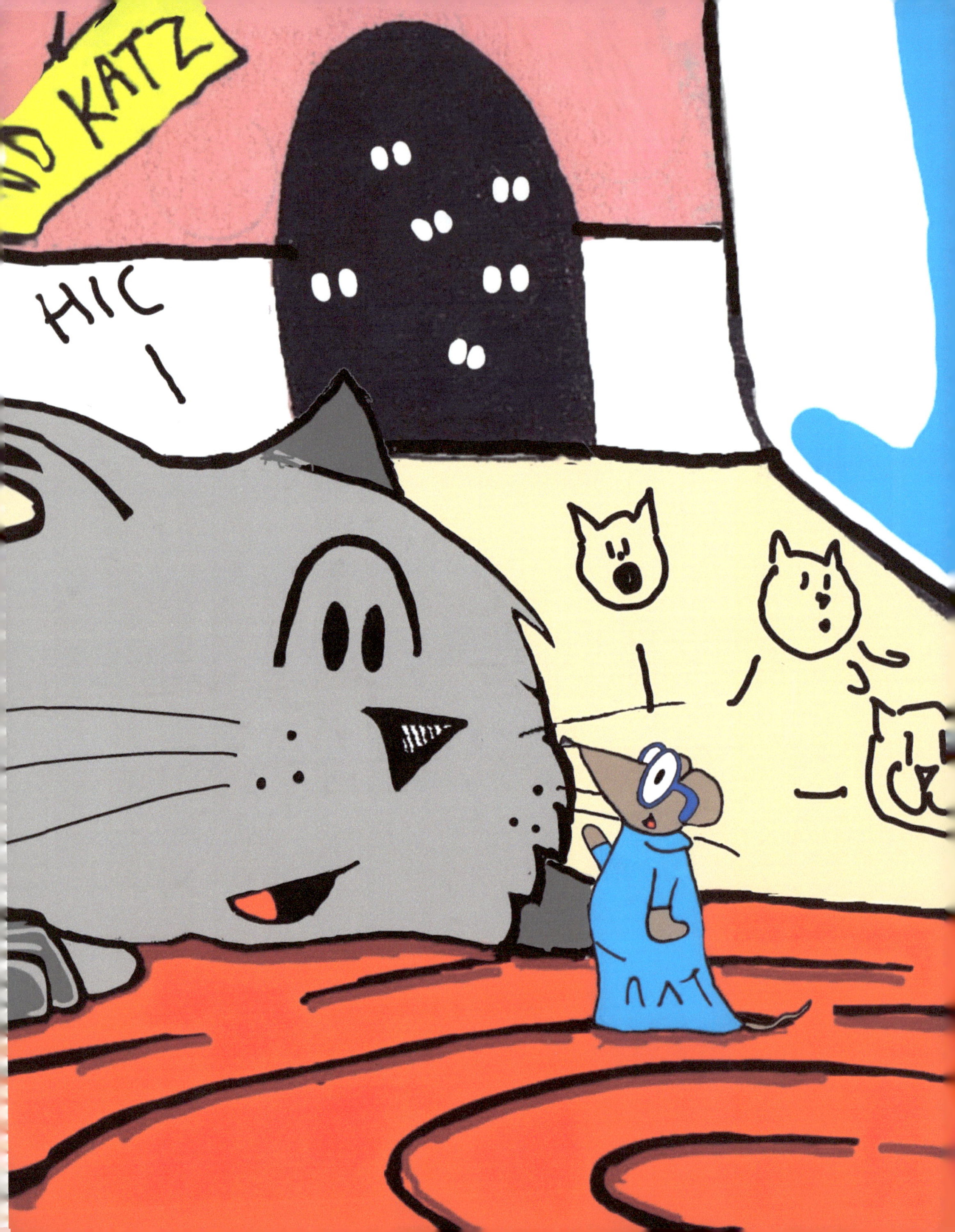

KATZ
HIC

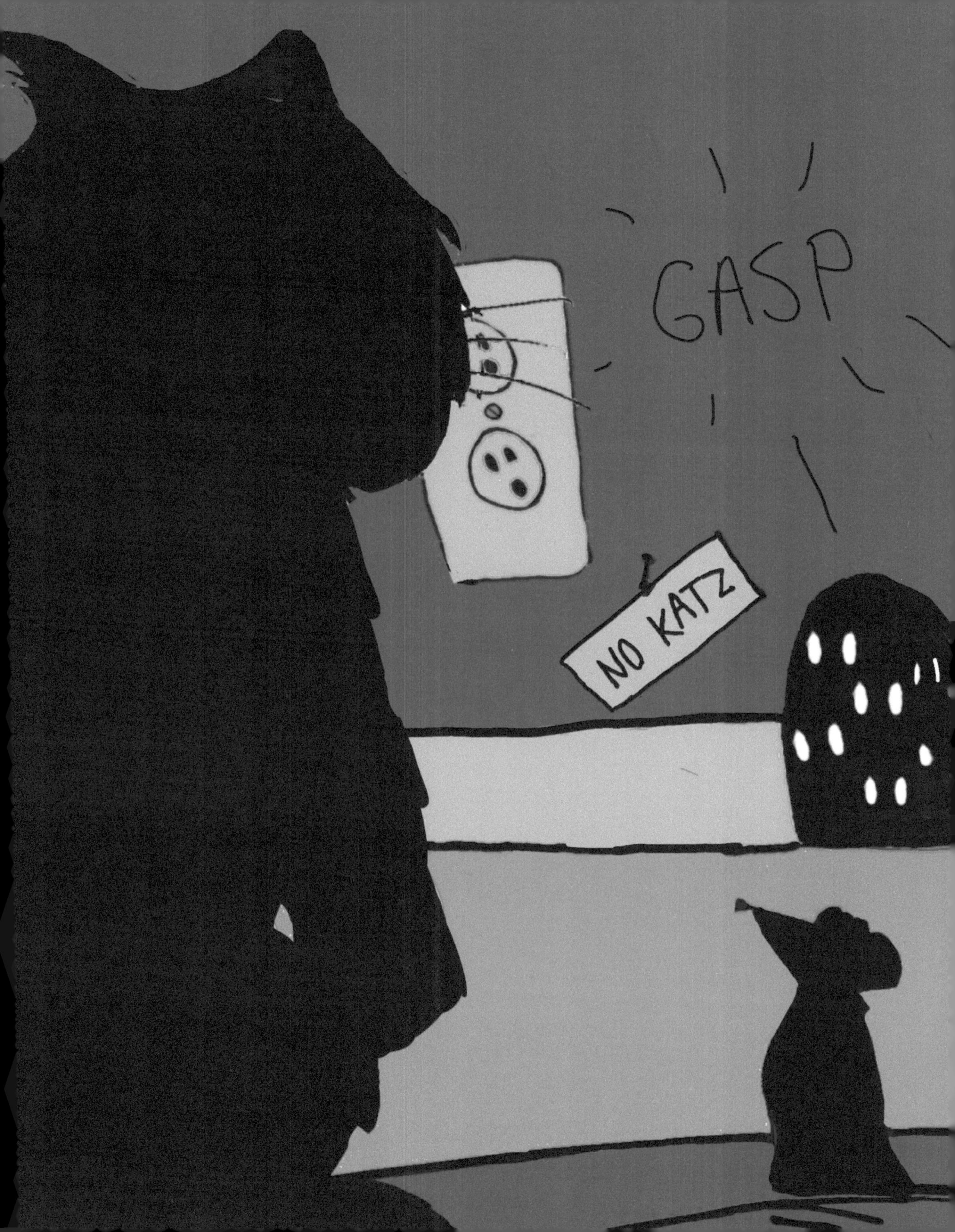

GASP
NO KATZ

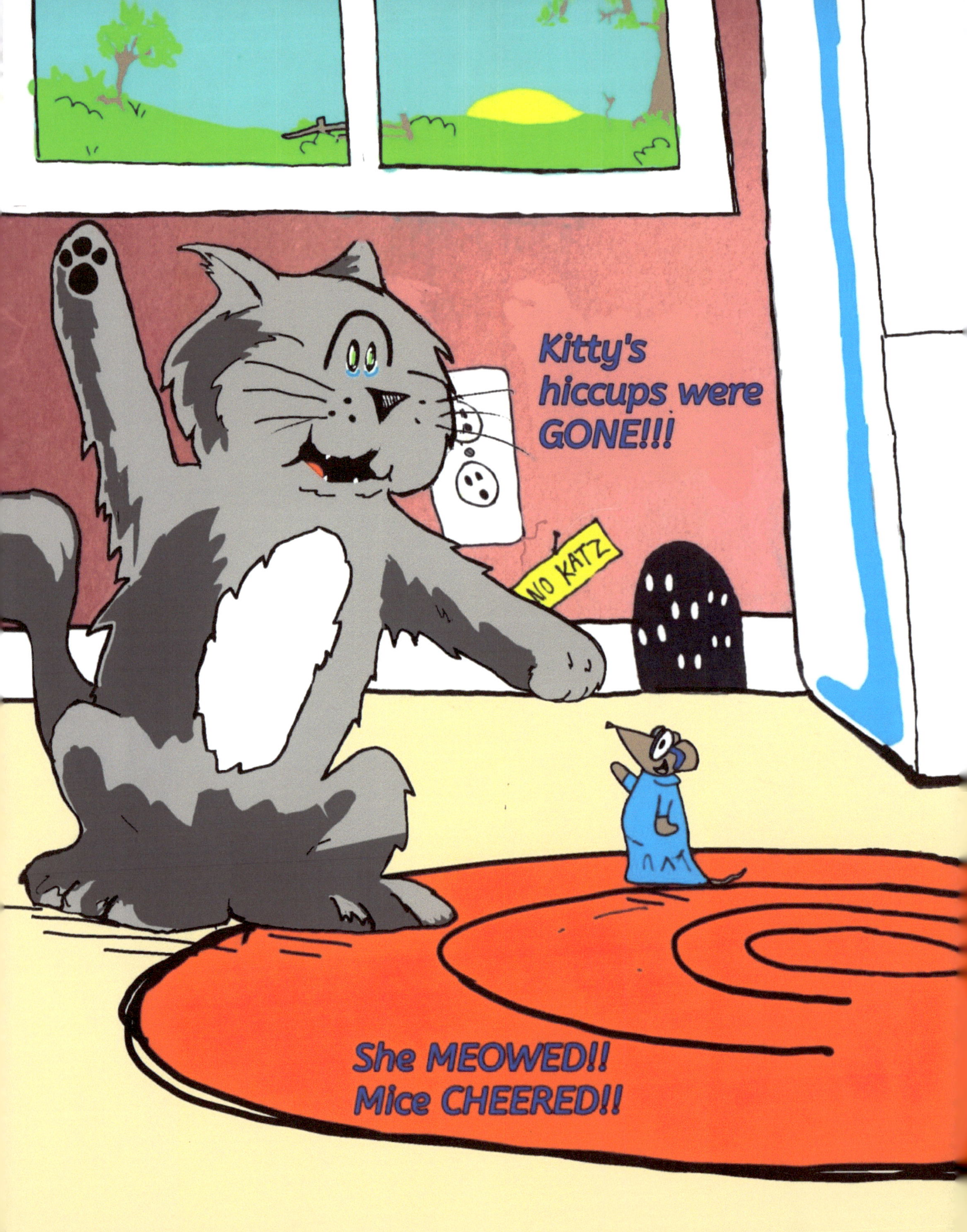

Kitty's hiccups were GONE!!!
NO KATZ
She MEOWED!! Mice CHEERED!!

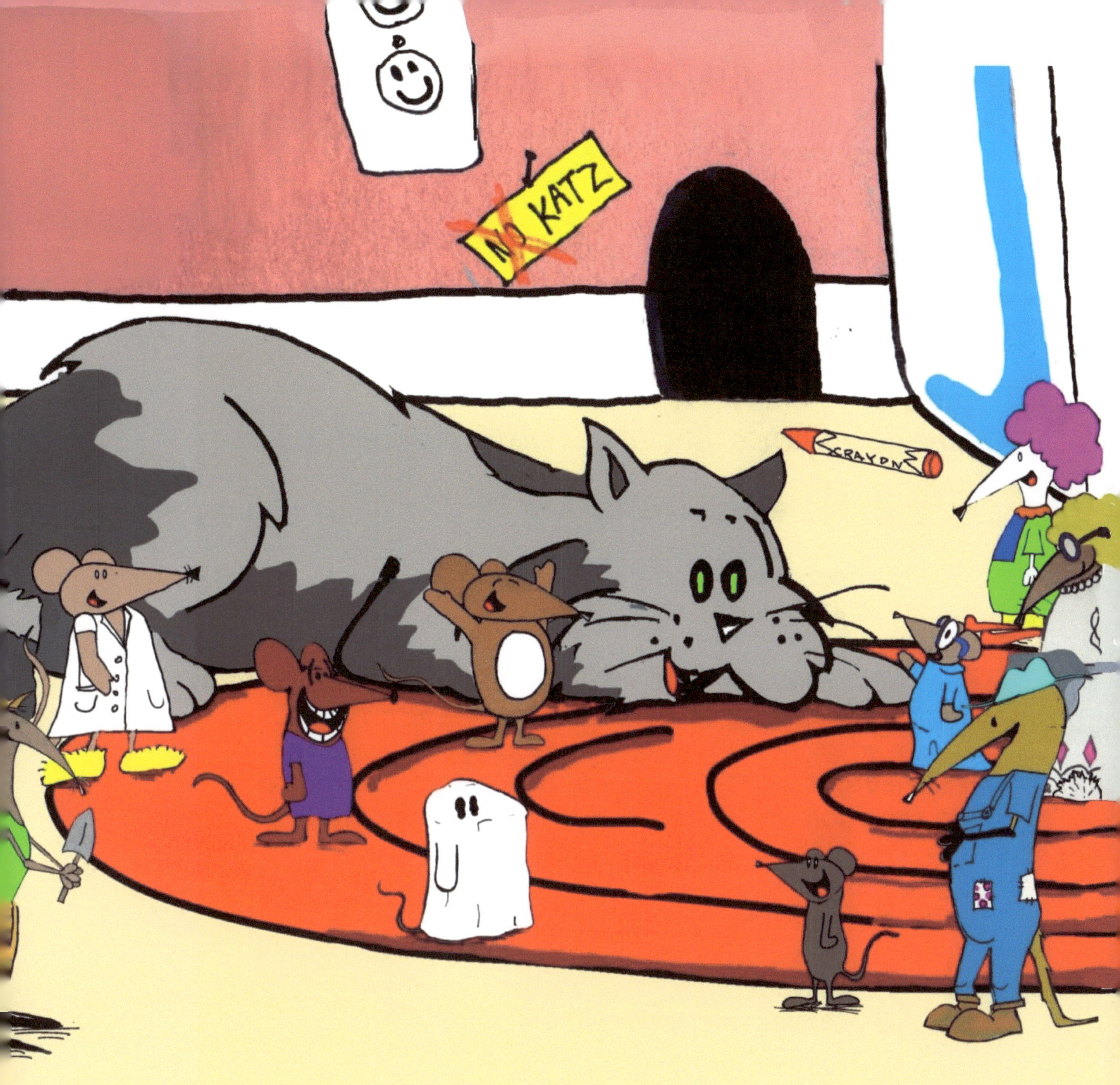

For kitties and hiccups were no longer feared!

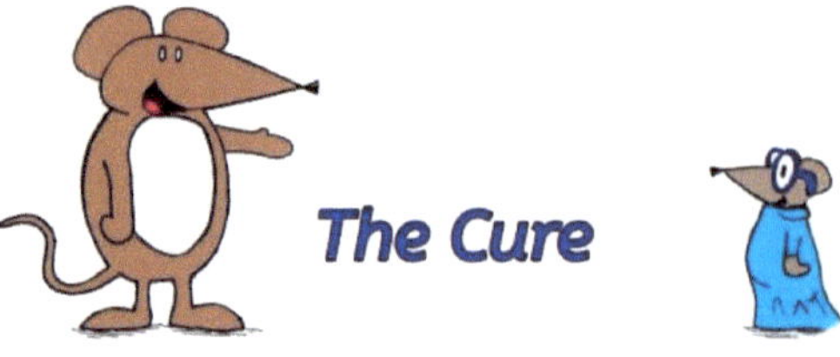

Time your hiccups,usually less than 10 seconds apart

Relax and take deep breaths and fill your lungs with oxygen

The moment the hiccup passes quickly inhale AS MUCH
AIR AS YOU CAN and KEEP YOUR AIRWAY OPEN.

Keep your lungs packed with air, breath in and out only
tiny tiny breaths if you need without releasing pressure.

If done right there won't be another hiccup, and once
the time you counted has passed gently let out the air.

If you release too fast or move quickly they will come back.
Relax for a moment and breath slow.

It may take additional tries, Relax. Don't get upset.
It will work and works best when somebody helps.

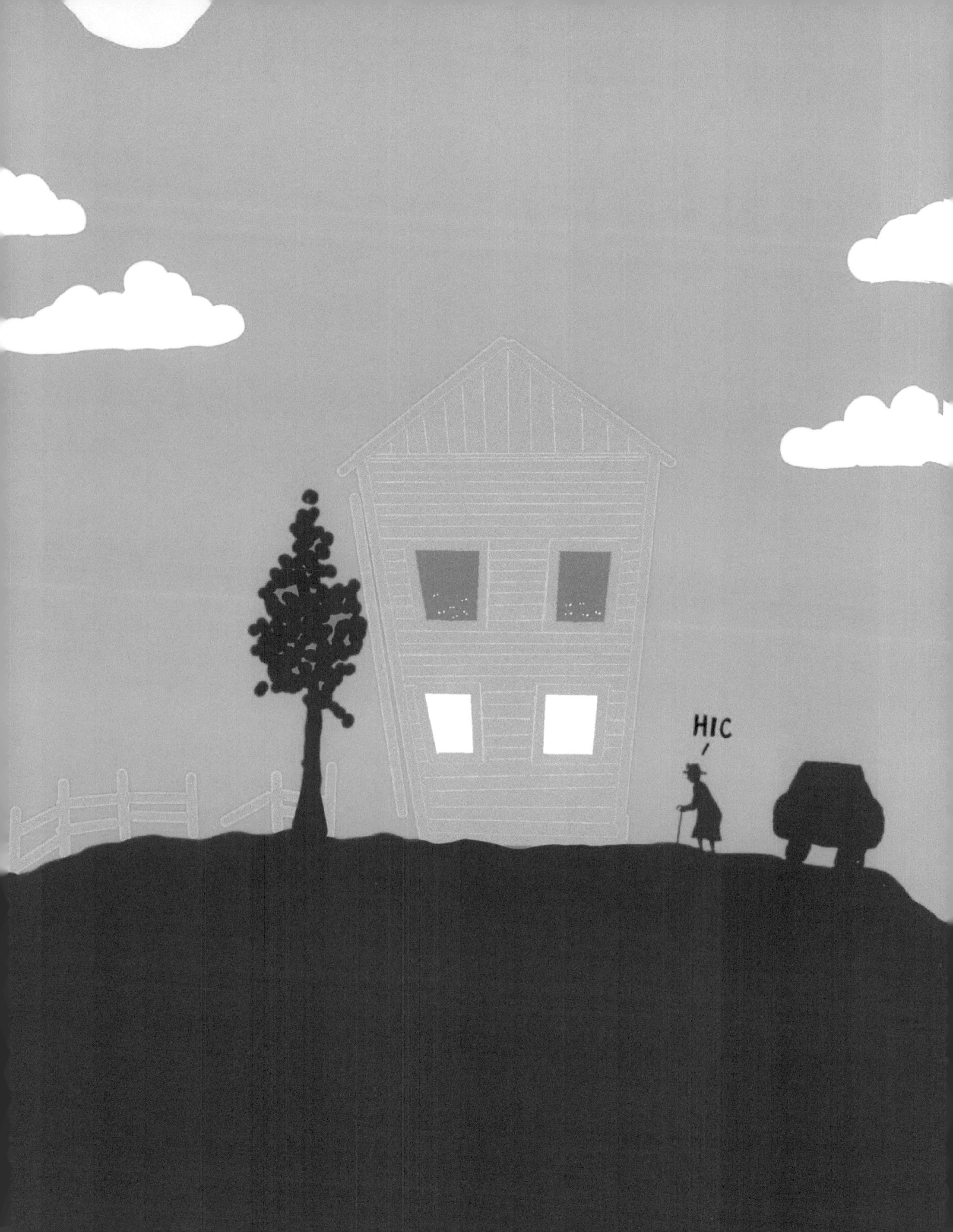
HIC